Birth Control

a woman's choice

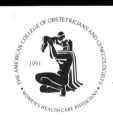

The American College
of Obstetricians and
Gynecologists
Women's Health Care Physicians

409 12th Street, SW
Washington, DC 20024-2188

Appreciation is extended to the following expert reviewers:

Philip A. Corfman, MD
Philip P. Darney, MD
Mitchell I. Edelson, MD
Phillip Stubblefield, MD
Lynda J. Wolf, MD

ACOG Staff:
Tatum Birdsall, Senior Editor
Barbara Gasque, Designer

Illustrations:
Terese Winslow

Library of Congress Cataloging-in-Publication Data
Birth control : a woman's choice.
p. cm.
Includes bibliographical references and index.
ISBN 0-915473-87-9 (pbk.: alk. paper)
1. Contraception--Popular works. 2. Birth control--Popular works.
[DNLM: 1. Contraception--methods--Popular Works. 2. Family
Planning--methods--Popular Works. WP 630 B6185 2003] I. American
College of Obstetricians and Gynecologists.
RG136.2.B55 2003
613.9'4--dc21
2002008314

Designed as an aid to patients, *Birth Control: A Woman's Choice* sets forth
current information and opinions on subjects related to women's health
and reproduction. The information does not dictate an exclusive course of
treatment or procedure to be followed and should not be construed as
excluding other medical opinions or acceptable methods of practice.
Variations taking into account the needs of the individual patient,
resources, and limitations unique to the institution or type of practice may
be appropriate.

12345/76543

Contents

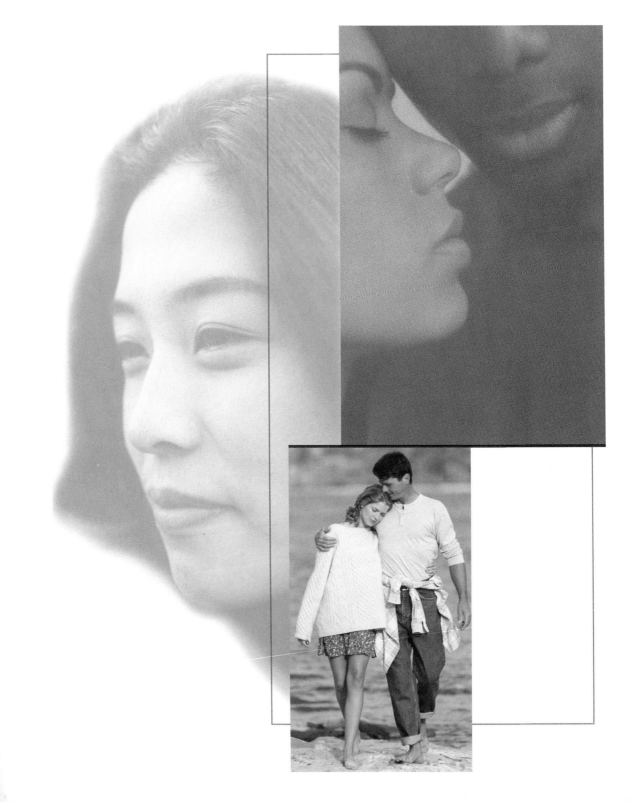

Preface

Birth control is an important issue for women for many years of their lives. From their early teens until their 40s, most women can become pregnant. Despite the availability of birth control, about half of all pregnancies are unplanned.

Birth control can help you plan the right time to have—or not have—a baby. Family planning is important to your health and the health of your children. Some methods of birth control also have other benefits, such as helping prevent **sexually transmitted diseases** and other health problems.

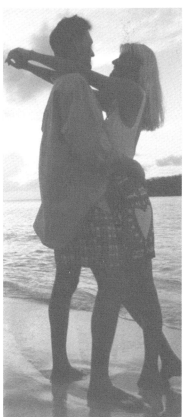

Today, there are many choices of birth control for women and men (see Appendix). No one method of birth control is right for every person.

Your decision to use a certain birth control method should be based on a number of factors. Some of these may include:

- Your age

- Your interest in having children later (Do you want to be able to stop using it at any time to become pregnant? Do you want a method of birth control that will last the rest of your fertile life?)

- Your cultural and religious beliefs

- Your need to protect yourself against sexually transmitted diseases

- Your preferences and your partner's preferences

- How well the method works

- Convenience and how likely you are to use it (Will you use it if you have to put it in place every time you have sex? Will you use it if you're in a hurry? Are you comfortable touching your body to put it in place?)

- Your ability to use the method successfully

- Risks and side effects

- Noncontraceptive benefits of the method

- How much it costs, month by month and over time

- How often you have intercourse

There are many factors to consider when choosing the method that best meets your needs. This book is designed to help you select the method of birth control that is best for you.

Reproduction

The Basics of Reproduction

Knowing the basics of reproduction will help you understand how birth control works. The more you know, the easier it will be to choose a method that's right for you.

The Female Reproductive System

Almost all of a woman's reproductive system is in her pelvis (see figure). The uterus, which is in the lower abdomen, opens into the vagina. A woman has two ovaries, one on each side of the uterus. The ovaries contain eggs. The ovaries are connected to the uterus by a pair of ducts called the fallopian tubes.

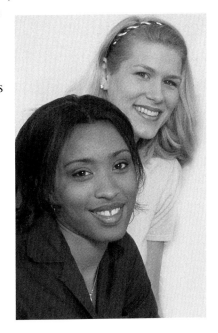

The outside of the female genital area is called the vulva. The fleshy part of this area that lies directly over the joint of the pubic bone is called the mons. The outer lips of the vulva are called the labia majora. The inner lips are called the labia minora. The clitoris is at the top of the inner lips. For most women, the clitoris is a center of sexual pleasure. It is partly covered by a fold of tissue called the hood. The perineum is the area between the anus and the *vagina*. The vestibule is found within the inner lips. The vagina and the urethra open

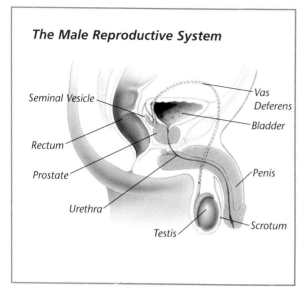

The Male Reproductive System

Seminal Vesicle

Rectum

Prostate

Urethra

Testis

Vas Deferens

Bladder

Penis

Scrotum

into the vestibule. Just inside the vestibule are the openings to the glands that make lubrication.

The Male Reproductive System

Much of a man's reproductive system is external (see figure). Sperm are tiny cells made in a man's *testes* in the sac (scrotum) below his penis. When the sperm cells mature, they leave the testes through small tubes called the *vas deferens*, or vas. These tubes carry the sperm to a larger tube in the *penis* called the *urethra*. As sperm travel through the vas, they mix with fluid from the *seminal vesicles* and the *prostate gland*, small organs located near the bladder. This mixture of sperm and fluid is called semen.

How Pregnancy Occurs

A woman's fertility depends on her menstrual cycle. Changes that occur during each cycle are caused by hormones—substances made by your body to control certain functions. Each month, hormones direct your uterus to build up a lining of blood-rich tissue (endometrium). These hormones also send a signal for an egg to ripen in a follicle—one of the tiny, fluid-filled sacs in your ovaries. When the egg is ripe, it's released from the ovary and moves into a fallopian tube. This process is called ovulation.

Signs that you may be ovulating include:

- A twinge or cramp, called mittelschmerz—or "middle pain"—in your lower abdomen or back

- Breast tenderness

- Increase in cervical mucus (vaginal discharge)

In a woman with a regular menstrual cycle, ovulation occurs 12–14 days before the start of her next menstrual period. A woman can get pregnant if she has unprotected sex with a man around the time of ovulation.

The average menstrual cycle lasts about 28 days, counting from the first day of one period (day 1) to the first day of the next. Cycles ranging from as few as 23 days to as many as 35 days are normal. Your own cycle may vary somewhat from month to month. By keeping a menstrual calendar for a few months, you can get an idea of what is normal for you.

After you have ovulated, the egg moves through one of the fallopian tubes to your uterus. If it isn't fertilized by a man's sperm, the egg dissolves. The levels of hormones then decrease. This signals the lining of the uterus to shed. This shedding is your monthly period.

During sex, when the man ejaculates (climaxes), semen travels out through the urethra in the penis and into the woman's vagina. Millions of sperm are deposited in a woman's vagina.

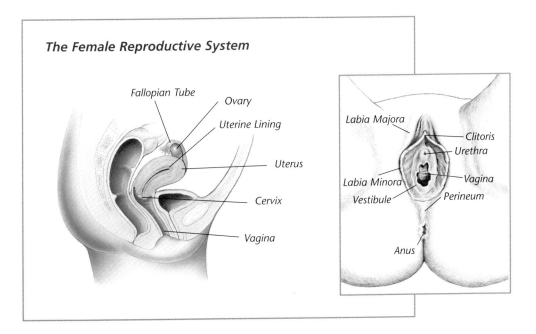

The Female Reproductive System

Fallopian Tube
Ovary
Uterine Lining
Uterus
Cervix
Vagina

Labia Majora
Clitoris
Urethra
Labia Minora
Vagina
Vestibule
Perineum
Anus

The Menstrual Cycle

Day 1

The first day of your menstrual period is considered day 1 of your cycle.

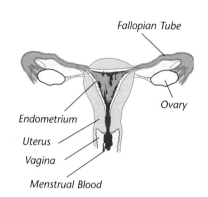

Day 5

The hormone estrogen signals the endometrium to grow and thicken.

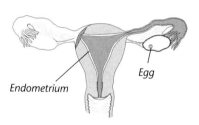

Day 14

An egg is released from the ovary and moves into one of the two fallopian tubes.

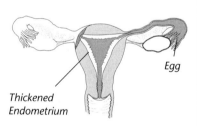

Day 28

If the egg is not fertilized, hormone levels decrease, and the endometrium is shed during menstruation.

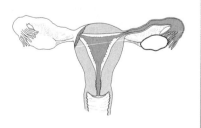

Hormones

Hormones are chemicals that control when and how certain organs work. They are made by glands in the body. The menstrual cycle and pregnancy are controlled by key hormones that interact at various stages:

- *Estrogen* and *progesterone:* Produced by the ovaries, these hormones trigger changes in the endometrium, causing it to thicken during each menstrual cycle and to shed if pregnancy does not occur. After an egg is fertilized, a sharp increase in these hormones keeps you from ovulating and having your period. During menopause, the ovaries stop making enough estrogen to thicken the lining of the uterus. This is when the menstrual periods stop.

- Follicle-stimulating hormone and luteinizing hormone: These hormones are made by the pituitary gland, a small organ located at the base of the brain. Follicle-stimulating hormone causes eggs to mature. Luteinizing hormone causes them to be released by the ovaries.

- Gonadotropin-releasing hormone: This hormone, also made in the brain, tells the pituitary gland when to produce follicle-stimulating hormone and luteinizing hormone.

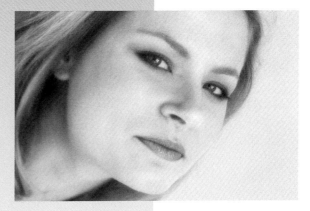

- Human chorionic gonadotropin: This hormone is produced during pregnancy. Made by certain cells from the fertilized and quickly dividing egg, human chorionic gonadotropin causes increases in estrogen and progesterone during pregnancy. It is the hormone that is detected in a pregnancy test.

The sperm travel up through the *cervix*, through the uterus, and out into the tubes.

Sperm can live inside a woman's body for 3 days or more. An egg's life span, though, is short: 12–24 hours. If an egg is waiting in a fallopian tube when a man ejaculates into the vagina, or if one is released during the next few days, it can be fertilized. The fertilized egg then moves down the fallopian tube to the uterus. It attaches to the lining of the uterus and grows into a *fetus*. The box illustrates this process.

The Reproductive Process

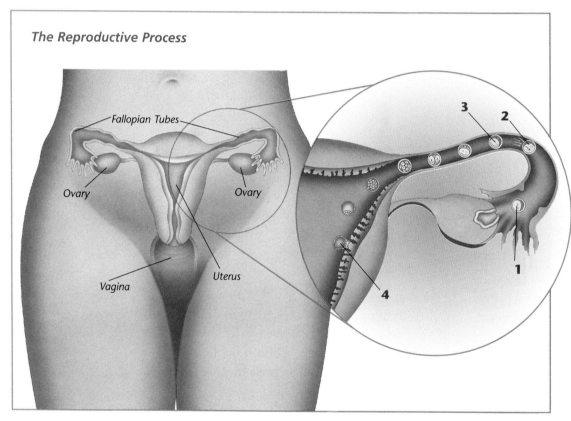

Each month during ovulation an egg is released (1) and moves into one of the fallopian tubes (2). If a woman has sex around this time, an egg may meet a sperm in the fallopian tube, and the two will join (3). This is called fertilization. The fertilized egg then moves through the fallopian tube into the uterus and may attach there to grow during pregnancy (4).

Fertility

For young, healthy couples not using birth control, the odds are about 25% that a woman will conceive during any one menstrual cycle. This figure starts to decrease in a woman's late 20s and early 30s and decreases even more after age 35 years. A man's fertility also declines with age, but not as early as most women's fertility.

If you are not using birth control, the length of time it takes to become pregnant will depend on several factors, such as:

- Your age
- Your health
- How often you have sex
- When you have sex

Most couples conceive within 6 months of having regular sex without birth control. Almost all (85 out of 100) are pregnant within a year. The remaining 15% may have fertility problems. Couples who want children and have not been able to conceive after 12 months of having regular sex should talk with their doctor (See "Infertility Treatment," under "Pregnancy Choices").

Why Use Birth Control?

As a woman grows and changes during her life, she may have different reasons for using birth control. Some women may not want to get pregnant, whereas others may want protection from sexually transmitted diseases (STDs). Certain methods of birth control offer health benefits as well as prevent pregnancy.

Pregnancy Prevention

Most women can become pregnant from the onset of menstruation until around the time that *menopause* begins. For most women, this is from their early teens until their 40s. About half of all pregnancies are unplanned. Birth control helps a

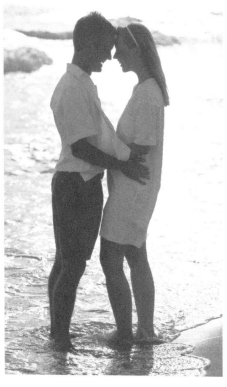

woman prevent an unwanted pregnancy. It can also help her plan a pregnancy. It can help her space the birth of her children and allows her to decide when it is best to have them.

If you have a baby, you need to think about birth control right after the birth. You may even want to discuss birth control options with your doctor while you are pregnant. Even if you want your children to be close in age, it's best to wait at least 18 months before getting pregnant again. It is unclear why the longer time between pregnancies may affect fetal health. It is believed that women who conceive babies fewer than 6 months (or more than 10 years) after birth have a higher risk of *preterm birth* and smaller babies. Babies born soon after their siblings may have problems because the woman's body has not had time to recover from the previous pregnancy. Postpartum (after delivery) stress also may be a factor. Some women may need to recover emotionally after the birth of a child.

Each family has different needs and desires when it comes to child spacing. Discuss the issue with your partner and your doctor.

If you are not breastfeeding, you may ovulate within weeks of giving birth. If you are breastfeeding, it may take longer for ovulation to return. It can be hard to tell when fertility returns because a woman can ovulate (and get pregnant) without having a period. Keep in mind, too, that if you used fertility drugs to conceive your baby, it doesn't mean that you can't get pregnant without them.

Sexually Transmitted Disease Prevention

Sexually transmitted diseases are infections that are spread by sexual contact. Anyone who has sexual contact with another person can get an STD.

You are at higher risk for STDs if you have had more than one sexual partner or if your partner has had more than one sexual partner. Use of condoms can help prevent some STDs. Condoms can be used along with other birth control methods, such as the pill or injections.

Types of STDs include:

- Chlamydial infection, which can damage the fallopian tubes and cause scarring, *pelvic inflammatory disease, infertility,* and problems during pregnancy.

- Gonorrhea, which may lead to pelvic inflammatory disease, infertility, and arthritis.

- Human papillomavirus, the common name for a group of related viruses. Some of these viruses cause genital warts and some are linked to cervical changes and cervical cancer.

- Genital herpes, which is caused by a virus that produces painful, highly infectious sores on or around the sex organs.

- Human immunodeficiency virus (HIV), a virus that attacks certain cells of the body's *immune system* and causes *acquired immunodeficiency syndrome (AIDS).*

- Syphilis, which is caused by an organism called *Treponema pallidum* and may cause major health problems or death in its later stages.

Condoms are the only method of birth control that protect against HIV.

Prevention is the key to fighting STDs (see box). Sexually transmitted diseases can cause severe damage to your body—even death. Even if there are no symptoms, a person with an STD can pass it to others by contact with skin, genitals, mouth, rectum, or body fluids. If you think you have an STD, seek medical treatment to avoid long-term health problems.

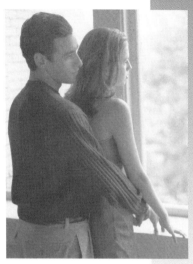

Protect Yourself

You can reduce the risk of STDs, including HIV, if you:

- Know your partner. It's not just your own behavior that puts you at risk for infection—it's your partner's, too. Ask about his sexual history and whether he has ever used intravenous drugs.

- Limit sexual partners. The more partners you or your partner(s) have, the higher the risk of getting an STD.

- Use a latex condom. Proper condom use helps protect you and your partner from infection with STDs.

- Avoid risky sex practices. Sexual acts that tear or break the skin carry a higher risk of STDs. Even small cuts that don't bleed let germs in and out. Anal sex poses a high risk because tissues in the rectum break easily. Oral sex also may pose a risk.

Other Benefits

Some methods of birth control offer health benefits in addition to preventing pregnancy. For instance, women who use birth control pills have a lower risk of cancer of the ovary and endometrium, benign (not cancer) breast disease, and *ectopic pregnancy.* The diaphragm lowers the risk of pelvic inflammatory disease and infertility, as well as the risk of some STDs. Some types of injections decrease the risk of cancer of the endometrium, recurrent yeast infections, and ectopic pregnancy.

Methods of Birth Control

Choosing a Method

Today, there are many choices of birth control for women and men. The more you know about birth control, the easier it will be to choose a method that meets your needs.

There are many different types of birth control:

- Barrier methods
  - —Spermicide
  - —Male and female condom
  - —Diaphragm
  - —Cervical cap
- Intrauterine device (IUD)
- Hormonal methods
  - —Combination birth control pill (oral contraceptive)
  - —*Progestin*-only pill
  - —Injection
  - —Vaginal ring
  - —Skin patch
  - —Emergency contraception
- Natural family planning
- Withdrawal

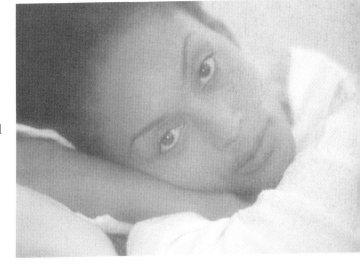

- Lactational *amenorrhea*
- Male and female sterilization

The diaphragm, cervical cap, IUD, birth control pill, injection, vaginal ring, and skin patch all require a prescription. Spermicides and condoms can be purchased over-the-counter. Even if you choose a method that does not need a prescription, you need to learn how to use it. A doctor, nurse, or family planning counselor can teach you.

More than one method may be used at the same time. For instance, using a condom with another method increases effectiveness and also protects against sexually transmitted diseases (STDs).

Birth control methods prevent pregnancy in a number of ways. They:

- Block the sperm from reaching the egg
- Kill sperm
- Keep eggs from being released each month
- Change the lining of the uterus
- Thicken the mucus in the cervix so that sperm can't easily pass through it

All methods of birth control have a chance of failure (see Table 1). But when a method is used correctly and every time you have sex, the failure rates are lower. Any method of birth control described here can work well if it is used the right way and is used each time you have sex.

Most women and couples use different methods over their lifetimes. At any given time, you may find that one method of birth control works better than others. For example, you may start to use a new method after the birth of a baby because some types of birth control can interfere with breastfeeding.

There are many different types of birth control. Each method has good points as well as *side effects*. Birth control allows a woman to plan her family—both the number and the spacing of children.

Table 1. Failure Rates for Methods of Birth Control*

Method	Percentage of Women with Pregnancy	
	Lowest Expected	Typical
No method	85.0	85.0
Spermicides	6.0	26.0
Periodic abstinence	—	25.0
Postovulation	1.0	—
Symptothermal	2.0	—
Ovulation method	3.0	—
Calendar	9.0	—
Cervical cap and spermicide		
Has not had a birth	9.0	20.0
Has had a birth	26.0	40.0
Diaphragm and spermicides	6.0	20.0
Withdrawal	4.0	19.0
Condom		
Female	5.0	21.0
Male	3.0	14.0
Birth control pill		5.0
Combination	0.1	—
Progestin-only	0.5	—
IUD		
Copper	0.6	0.8
Hormonal	0.1	0.1
Vaginal ring	1.0	N/A
Skin patch	1.0	N/A
Injections	0.3	0.3
Sterilization		
Female	0.5	0.5
Male	0.1	0.15

*Rates during first year of use, United States. Lowest expected percentages are based on perfect use, when the couple uses the method correctly every time they have sex. Typical percentages are based on use by a large group of people using the method, which will include incorrect or missed use.

Abbreviations: IUD, intrauterine device; N/A, not applicable.

Modified from Trussell J. Contraceptive efficacy. In: Hatcher RA, Trussell J, Stewart F, Cates W Jr, Stewart GK, Guest F, et al. Contraceptive technology. 17th revised edition. New York: Ardent Media, 1998:779–844

Barrier Methods

Barrier methods are among the oldest and safest forms of birth control. These methods work by acting as barriers to keep the man's sperm from reaching the woman's egg. Some methods also may protect against STDs.

The use of barrier methods goes back 3,500 years. Today, barrier methods are a safe and effective way to prevent pregnancy. The types of barrier methods used in the United States include spermicide, condom (male and female), diaphragm, cervical cap, and Lea's Shield.

Another type of barrier method is the sponge. Although it is not currently on the market, it was once available for sale in the United States and may be again in the future. The sponge is a doughnut-shaped device made of a soft foam that is coated with spermicide. It is pushed up in the vagina to cover the cervix. It acts as a physical and chemical barrier between the sperm and the cervix.

Spermicides are chemical barriers. The other methods are physical barriers. Combining spermicides with physical barrier methods provides more protection. Some barrier methods— such as the diaphragm, cervical cap, and Lea's shield—rely on spermicide for their full effectiveness and should be used with each act of sex.

Barrier methods are not as effective as some other birth control methods, such as birth control pills or the IUD. When two barrier methods are used together (such as a diaphragm and a condom), they become a highly effective form of birth control.

Most of the time, barrier methods have no side effects on other systems in your body. However, if either you or your partner is allergic to latex, do not use a barrier method that contains rubber or latex. It may cause a reaction in your body.

Barrier methods are most effective when used the correct way every time you have sex. Even one act of sex without birth control can result in pregnancy. If your barrier method breaks or becomes dislodged, you may want to consider emergency contraception.

Spermicides

Spermicides are chemical barriers. They include:

- Tablets
- Foam
- Cream
- Jelly
- Film (thin sheets that contain spermicide)

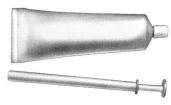

Spermicide

How They Work

Spermicides contain a chemical that kills sperm or makes them not active. As a result, the sperm cannot pass through the woman's cervix and fertilize an egg.

Lea's Shield

The Lea's Shield is a dome-shaped silicone device with a loop for removal that fits inside the woman's vagina and covers her cervix. It is a barrier method of birth control and is used with spermicide.

The Lea's Shield comes in only one size and requires a prescription. It has a one-way valve that lets secretions flow out without letting sperm in.

The Lea's Shield can be inserted hours before sexual intercourse. However, it must be left in place for at least 8 hours after intercourse, but should not be in place for more than 48 hours total. It can be reused and should be washed with soap and water between uses. This device does not protect against STDs.

Because the Lea's Shield was just recently approved for use by the U.S. Food and Drug Administration, there are limited data available on its use. A total of 9–14 per 100 women get pregnant while using this method.

How to Use Them

Spermicides are easy to use. They are low cost and can be bought over-the-counter.

Spermicides are placed in the vagina before each act of sex. Spermicides can be used with condoms, and they are applied to a diaphragm or cervical cap before it is inserted. They must be reapplied for each act of sex. Be sure to follow the instructions supplied with the product. Use the applicator that comes with it.

Some spermicides are not effective right away. For instance, films and tablets must be placed in the vagina 10–30 minutes before sex. They require time to melt and become active.

Side Effects and Risks

When spermicides are used alone, as many as 1 in 4 women become pregnant while using this method. Spermicides are most effective when used with another barrier method. They are not linked to any increased risk for birth defects if you become pregnant.

The risk of a urinary tract problems or vaginitis may be increased with the use of spermicides. Excessive use may cause vaginal irritation.

Male Condom

A male condom is a thin sheath made of latex (rubber), polyurethane (plastic), or animal membrane. It is worn by the man over the erect penis. Condoms do not cost very much. They are available over-the-counter in many supermarkets, drug stores, and other stores, so they are easy to find and buy.

Many types of condoms are available. Some condoms may even come in different shapes, sizes, and colors. Some may have shaped ends that provide a place to hold the semen. They are sold either dry or lubricated. Some contain spermicide. Only water-based lubricants should be used with condoms. Oil can damage them. Condoms should be stored away from heat and light.

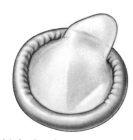

Male Condom

Of all birth control methods, latex condoms provide the best protection against STDs, including human immunodeficiency virus (HIV). Condoms made of animal membrane do not protect against STDs as well as those made of latex.

How It Works

The male condom acts as a physical barrier to keep the sperm from entering the cervix and getting to the egg. When sperm is released, it stays inside the condom and does not pass into the woman's vagina.

How to Use It

A condom should be used only once and only one should be used at a time. Although condoms are simple to use, to be effective they must be used correctly throughout each act of sex (see box). They can be used with other methods of birth control to increase effectiveness.

Side Effects and Risks

Condoms may blunt sensation for the man and the woman. Like some other barrier methods, they must be used with each act of sex.

About 1 in 7 women who use condoms without spermicide become pregnant. This rate can vary greatly, depending on how well they are used.

How to Use a Male Condom

To use the male condom, place the rolled-up condom over the tip of the erect penis. Hold the end of the condom to allow a little extra space at the tip. Then unroll the condom over the penis.

Right after ejaculation, grasp the condom around the base of the penis as it is withdrawn. Throw the condom away. It should never be reused.

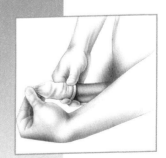

Some people are allergic to latex. These people might consider using condoms made from animal membrane or plastic. Remember, though, that condoms made from animal membrane do not provide the same protection against STDs.

Female Condom

The female condom is a thin plastic pouch that lines the vagina. It is held in place by a closed inner ring at the cervix and an outer ring at the opening of the vagina. It is best suited for women whose partners will not use a male condom.

Female condoms can be used with other methods of birth control to increase effectiveness. They can be bought over-the-counter and do not need to be fitted. They cost more than male condoms.

Some couples prefer the female condom to the male condom. The female condom conducts heat better than the male condom. It does not feel tight around the penis. Female condoms may provide some protection against STDs.

How It Works

The female condom provides a physical barrier that prevents sperm from entering the cervix. Like the male condom, the female condom is more effective when used with a spermicide.

How to Use It

The female condom is inserted much like a diaphragm (see "Diaphragm" and box, "How to Use a Condom"). It comes with a lubricant. You can use both oil- and water-based lubricants with it. The female condom can be inserted up to 8 hours before sex.

Female condoms should be used only once. They are difficult to insert and require careful use. Sex may be noisy if not enough lubrication is used.

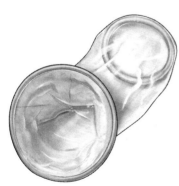

Female Condom

How to Use a Female Condom

To use the female condom, squeeze the inner ring between your fingers and insert it into the vagina as far as possible. Push the inner ring up until it is just behind the pubic bone. About an inch of the open end should be outside your body.

Right after ejaculation, squeeze and twist the outer ring and pull the pouch out gently. Throw the condom away. It should never be reused.

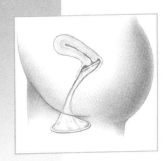

A female condom should not be used with a male condom. It puts both condoms at increased risk of breakage.

Side Effects and Risks

Almost 1 in 5 women who use the female condom for birth control become pregnant. There are no other side effects or risks.

Diaphragm

The diaphragm is a small round rubber dome that fits inside the woman's vagina and covers her cervix. It is used with a spermicide.

A diaphragm requires a prescription. Diaphragms come in a range of sizes (diameter of the rim). You will need to see a doctor or nurse to be fitted. Women should be fitted with the largest comfortable size. To use a diaphragm, a woman's vaginal muscles must be able to hold it in place.

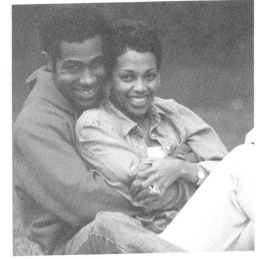

After you are fitted, you will be shown how to insert and remove the diaphragm. You also will learn how to check if it is placed properly and how to care for it (see box).

You will need to be refitted if:

- You gain or lose 10 pounds or more

- You have had pelvic surgery

- You have repeated urinary tract infections

- You or your partner feel pain or pressure during sex

- You give birth or have a *miscarriage*

For most women, it is easier to insert a diaphragm than a cervical cap. The cost is fairly low. A diaphragm should be replaced with a new one about every 2 years.

Using the diaphragm reduces the risk of some STDs. When the diaphragm is used with the male condom, it provides added protection from pregnancy and STDs.

How It Works

The diaphragm is a physical barrier that blocks the sperm from entering the cervix. The spermicide used with it kills sperm.

How to Use It

The diaphragm may be put in place up to 6 hours before you have sex. There are three basic steps to insert your diaphragm:

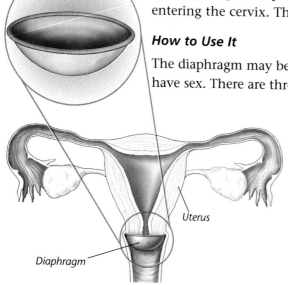

Uterus

Diaphragm

1. Apply spermicidal cream or jelly around the rim and inside the dome of the diaphragm. The spermicide must be on the side of the diaphragm facing or in contact with the cervix. It also can be put on both sides.

2. Squeeze the rim of the diaphragm between your fingers and insert it into your vagina. When the

diaphragm is pushed up as far as it will go, the front part of the rim should be up behind a bone you can feel in front of your pelvis (the pubic bone). Tuck the front rim of the diaphragm up as far as it will comfortably go.

3. Check to see if your cervix is covered. To do this, reach inside and touch your cervix. The cervix feels something like the tip of your nose. If you have trouble finding your cervix, talk with your doctor or nurse about how to place

Caring for Your Diaphragm

To remove the diaphragm, pull gently on the front rim. To wash the diaphragm, use mild soap and water. Rinse the soap off well (soap can damage the rubber), dry it, and put it back in its case.

A diaphragm may fade or change colors over time. It still can be used unless you notice holes in the rubber. Check your diaphragm for holes monthly. To check for holes, hold the diaphragm up to a light and stretch the rubber gently between your fingers. Filling the diaphragm with water also is a good way to check for holes.

Use only water-based lubricants when you use a diaphragm. Do not use any oil-based lubricants such as petroleum jelly or body lotion. The oil can damage the rubber. Do not use talcum powder to dry your diaphragm. Talc may increase the risk of ovarian cancer.

Have your diaphragm checked at your routine exam each year. Also have your diaphragm checked if it begins slipping out of place or if you have had pelvic surgery, have been pregnant, or have gained or lost at least 10 pounds. You may need to be fitted for a new size.

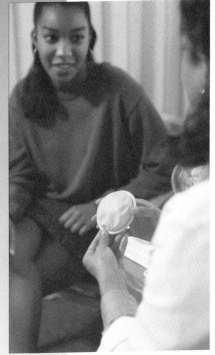

the diaphragm. After the diaphragm is in place, the cervix should be completely covered by the rubber dome.

A diaphragm is not effective without a spermicide. If you have inserted the diaphragm more than 2 hours before you have sex, you must insert a fresh supply of spermicide into the vagina just before you have sex. You must add more spermicide before each act of sex, no matter how closely timed they are. To do this, insert the spermicide into your vagina while the diaphragm is still in place. An applicator comes with the spermicidal cream or jelly.

The diaphragm may slip out of place, so be sure to check placement of it before and after sex. If the diaphragm is dislodged during sex, spermicide should be reapplied.

After sex, the diaphragm must be left in place for about 6 hours, but not more than 24 hours. It is important to take proper care of your diaphragm.

Side Effects and Risks

The failure rate for the diaphragm, when used with a spermicide, is 20%. The failure rates are higher in women who have had children.

A properly sized and fitted diaphragm should not cause pain or pressure to either you or your partner during sex. If it does, it may need to be refitted.

The diaphragm may increase the risk of urinary tract infections. If you get a urinary tract infection, your doctor may treat it with *antibiotics*. If you keep having infections, you may need to use a larger or smaller diaphragm. You may need to change to another type of birth control.

A diaphragm can cause irritation, or rarely, a systemic reaction to those who have an allergy to spermicide or latex. It cannot be used during menstruation or just after giving birth. Some women should not use a diaphragm (see box).

A Diaphragm Is Not an Option If You:

- Have poor vaginal or *perineal* muscle support or have certain forms of pelvic *prolapse*
- Have cervical abnormalities that prevent proper fitting
- Have a history of toxic shock syndrome
- Are not able to learn to insert and remove the device
- Have a history of high-blood-pressure reaction to the product or spermicides
- Have recurrent *cystitis*
- Have recurrent pelvic inflammatory disease

Cervical Cap

The cervical cap is a small thin rubber or plastic dome shaped like a thimble. It is smaller than a diaphragm. It fits tightly over the cervix and stays in place by suction.

Cervical caps come in four sizes. A doctor must prescribe and fit you for a cervical cap. You will then be taught how to insert and remove it.

Unlike the diaphragm, the cervical cap does not require strong vaginal muscles to use. It is less likely than the diaphragm to be felt by your partner during sex.

The cervical cap does have many similarities to the diaphragm, though:

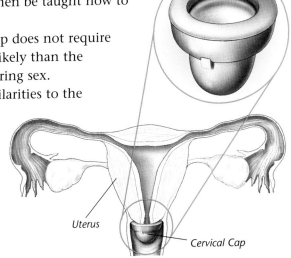

Uterus

Cervical Cap

- It is effective with consistent and correct use.
- It is low cost over the long term.
- It reduces the risk of some STDs
- Oil-based lubricants, such as petroleum jelly, should not be used with it.

- It may be used in combination with the male condom for better protection from pregnancy and STDs.
- It cannot be worn just after giving birth.
- It must be checked for wear or holes.
- It may need to be refitted after having a baby or after weight gain or loss.

Care for the cervical cap is similar to that of the diaphragm (see box, "Caring for Your Diaphragm"). A cervical cap needs to be replaced with a new one once a year.

How It Works

Like the diaphragm, the cervical cap works by blocking the sperm from entering the cervix. It also must be used with a spermicide. It differs from a diaphragm in that it can remain in place for up to 48 hours. Less spermicide is needed, and it does not need to be reapplied before each act of sex.

How to Use It

Inserting a cervical cap is a lot like inserting a diaphragm. Spermicide is placed inside the cap, which then is squeezed between your fingers and inserted into the vagina. The cap is then pressed onto the cervix until the cervix is completely covered. Before and after each act of sex, the cervix should be checked to make sure it is covered. This is done by pressing on the dome of the cap with your finger. After sex, the cap should be left in place for 6 hours but not longer than 48 hours.

Side Effects and Risks

When the cervical cap is used with a spermicide, about 1 in 5 women become pregnant. The failure rate is higher—about 2 in 5 women become pregnant—once a woman has had children.

The cervical cap sometimes causes irritation or odor in the vagina. This most often occurs if it is left in too long. It also may increase the risk of urinary tract infection. Some women cannot use the cervical cap (see box).

A Cervical Cap Is Not an Option If You:

- Cannot be fitted properly

- Have a history of toxic shock syndrome

- Are not able to learn to insert and remove the device

- Have an infection of the vagina or cervix

- Have known or suspected cancer of the uterus or cervix

- Have a history of high-blood-pressure reaction to the product or spermicides

Hormonal Methods

With hormonal birth control, a woman takes hormones similar to those her body makes naturally. In most cases, these hormones prevent ovulation. When there is no egg to be fertilized, pregnancy cannot occur. The hormones also cause other changes in the cervical mucus and uterus that help prevent pregnancy. Effective hormonal birth control comes in several forms:

- Birth control pills

  —Combination

  —Progestin-only

  —Emergency contraception

- Injections

- Vaginal ring

- Skin patch

Hormonal methods of birth control do not protect against STDs. Using condoms with them helps with this protection.

Combination Pills

Birth control pills are used by millions of women in the United States to prevent pregnancy. Most women who use hormonal birth control take the combination pill. It contains the hormones estrogen and progestin (a synthetic version of the hormone progesterone). There are many different brands with different doses of hormones. With such a variety, a woman can choose the pill that is right for her. Before your doctor or nurse will prescribe birth control pills for you, he or she will ask you some questions (see box) and may do a physical exam—which can include a pelvic exam and breast exam.

Taking the birth control pill is very effective. It is easy to use and convenient. You do not need to do anything else before sex to prevent pregnancy.

The pill does not affect a women's fertility after she stops taking it. If you could get pregnant before you took the pill, you still should be able to do so after you stop taking it. It may take you a little longer to get pregnant than if you had not been on the pill, though.

Many women have heard or believe things about the pill that aren't true. Table 2 lists some common myths and facts about the pill.

Women who are breastfeeding should not take the combination pill until milk flow is steady. Taking estrogen can cut down on their milk supply. Barrier methods—such as condoms—should be used until pill use is established. The progestin-only pill is a good choice for women who are breastfeeding because progestins increase milk production.

How They Work

The combination pill contains an estrogen and a progestin. These hormones, which are produced in the ovaries, affect the menstrual cycle and fertility. By altering the naturally occurring levels of these hormones, birth control pills can affect ovulation and other reproductive functions, such as the thickening of the cervical mucus and endometrium that occurs as a normal part of a woman's cycle.

Questions Your Doctor May Ask Before Prescribing the Pill

❏ How old are you?

❏ When was your last menstrual period?

❏ Do you have irregular or painful periods?

❏ Have you ever used birth control pills before?

❏ Have you ever used other types of birth control before? What types?

❏ Do you smoke?

❏ Have you ever had an STD?

❏ Have you had conditions or diseases such as breast cancer, blood clots, or stroke?

❏ Do you have a family history of any of these conditions?

❏ Do you take any medications?

❏ Do you have children? What were your pregnancies and deliveries like?

❏ Do you plan to have children in the future?

❏ Do you have any allergies?

❏ Have you ever had surgery?

❏ How many sexual partners do you have or have you had?

❏ What types of sexual behaviors do you practice?

Both estrogens and progestins cause the endometrium to change. When you are not pregnant, the level of progesterone decreases, the lining of the uterus is shed, and menstruation occurs. If you are pregnant, a sharp increase in these hormones keeps you from ovulating and having your period. Taking the

Table 2. Myths About the Pill

Myth	Fact
Taking the pill is risky.	The pill may be risky for women older than 35 years who smoke. For almost all women, though, the benefits of the pill outweigh any possible risks.
Taking the pill causes weight gain.	As many women lose weight as gain weight while taking the pill.
Taking a break from the pill now and then is a good idea.	There is no health benefit to taking a break from the pill. Taking a break may increase a woman's chances of an unwanted pregnancy.
The pill causes cancer.	Studies show that the pill does not increase the risk of cervical or breast cancer in most women. In fact, it decreases the risk of ovarian and endometrial cancer.
A woman will not be able to get pregnant unless she has stopped taking the pill for a long time.	The pill is out of a woman's system and she is able to get pregnant within 24 hours of when she stops taking it.

pill mimics this sharp increase enough to keep you from ovulating. Without an egg, pregnancy cannot occur. Because there are days when you do not take hormones, though, you still have your period, although it may be lighter, shorter, and more regular.

A backup is built into this system to provide protection if ovulation does occur. The hormones in the pill also cause changes in the cervical mucus and the endometrium. The cervical mucus thickens, blocking the sperm from entering the cervix. The endometrium thins, making it less likely that a fertilized egg can attach to the lining of the uterus. Together, these three events make it very unlikely that someone taking the pill will become pregnant.

How to Use Them

When you start taking the pill depends on the type of pill you are taking. You can start taking the pill on the first day of your period. You will not need a backup method of birth control. For convenience, many pill users start taking the pill on the Sunday after their periods start. You can start even if you are still bleeding. Women who start to take pills on a Sunday will have their periods in the middle of the week in most cases. Use another type of birth control for the next 7 days of the first cycle as a backup method. Condoms and foam (spermicides) are a good choice. This is the only time you will need to use a backup method unless you forget to take your pills.

Women who have had babies should talk to their doctor or nurse about when they can start the pill. The timing depends on whether they are breastfeeding. Women who have had a miscarriage or **abortion** can start taking the pill right away.

You will start each new pack of pills on the same day of the week as you started the first pack. It is a good idea to have an extra pack of pills and a backup method on hand in case you miss some pills or lose your pack.

Pills work only if you take them correctly. Do not skip pills for any reason—even if you bleed between periods or feel sick. Call your doctor or nurse if you are concerned. Even if you do not have sex very often, you should keep taking the pill.

Your pills may not work well if your body does not absorb them. This may happen if you are taking certain medications or if you vomit. If you can't keep your pill down, you should use a backup method for the rest of your cycle.

Pills come in packs of either 21 or 28 pills:

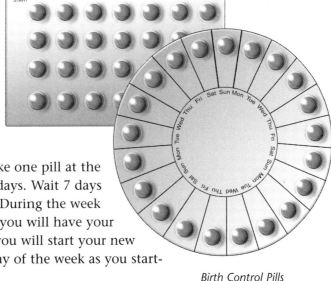

- If your pack has 21 pills, take one pill at the same time each day for 21 days. Wait 7 days before starting a new pack. During the week you are not taking the pill, you will have your period. Keep in mind that you will start your new pack of pills on the same day of the week as you started the first pack.

Birth Control Pills

- If your pack has 28 pills, take one pill at the same time each day for 28 days. When you finish all the pills in the pack, start a new pack the next day. During the week you are taking the last 7 pills, you will have your period.

Each new pack of pills comes with facts about the pill. Read this information and ask your doctor about anything that is not clear to you.

Health Benefits

The combination birth control pill has benefits in addition to preventing pregnancy. For instance, women who use the birth control pill have a lower risk of cancer of the endometrium and ovary. The pill also can help women achieve good cycle control. The box shows the health benefits of birth control pills.

The pill helps to keep your periods regular, lighter, and shorter and reduces menstrual cramps. It also lowers your risk of ectopic pregnancy (see box). Some types of birth control pills also can help treat acne.

Side Effects and Risks

The pill must be prescribed by a doctor. It is a very effective form of birth control. When women use the pill correctly, fewer than 1 in 100 will get pregnant over 1 year. However, about 3 in 100 typical users (3%) will become pregnant. A woman may get pregnant if a pill is missed or is not absorbed. If a dose is missed or not absorbed (because of vomiting, for instance), a backup method of birth control should be used (see box).

Some women have side effects when they are on the pill. These may include:

- Headache
- Tender breasts
- Nausea
- Irregular bleeding

Health Benefits of Combination Birth Control Pills

Besides being a highly effective method of birth control, birth control pills reduce the risk of:

- Cancer of the endometrium

- Ovarian cysts

- Pelvic inflammatory disease

- Acne

- Bone loss

- Benign breast disease

- Symptoms of polycystic ovary syndrome

- Premature ovarian failure

- Pain related to endometriosis

- *Breakthrough bleeding* in women taking blood thinners (anticoagulants)

- Iron-deficiency *anemia*

- Menstrual cycle irregularities

- *Dysmenorrhea*

- Heavy uterine bleeding

- Ectopic pregnancy

- Chronic *anovulation*

- Missed periods

- Depression

Side effects often go away after a few months of use. There will likely be fewer side effects if the pill is taken at the same time every day.

For nausea, many women find that taking the pill with a meal or before bed helps. For headaches, taking over-the-counter products for pain relief often helps.

Missing a period is common. If you miss one period and have taken the pill as prescribed, you should keep taking the pill. If you have forgotten some pills and miss one period, call your doctor. Don't stop taking the pill. It is not likely that you are pregnant. Using birth control pills during pregnancy does not increase the risk birth defects.

Ectopic Pregnancy

Sometimes the fertilized egg doesn't reach the uterus. It begins to grow in the fallopian tube or, rarely, attaches to an ovary or other organ in the abdomen. This is called an ectopic pregnancy. Because it is outside the uterus, an ectopic pregnancy cannot grow as it should and must be treated. About 1 in 60 pregnancies is ectopic.

Almost all ectopic pregnancies occur in the fallopian tube. Because the tube is so narrow and its wall is so thin, the pregnancy can grow to only about the size of a walnut before the tube bursts. This can occur anytime in the first 3 months of pregnancy. Because the tube may burst and cause major bleeding, ectopic pregnancy must be treated promptly once it is found.

Ectopic pregnancies can be hard to diagnose. Some women may have no symptoms at all and may not even know they are pregnant. The symptoms of ectopic pregnancy sometimes include the symptoms of pregnancy.

Other symptoms may include:

- Vaginal bleeding
- Abdominal pain
- Shoulder pain
- Weakness, dizziness, or fainting

Because an ectopic pregnancy can occur without warning, you should call your doctor right away about any pain or bleeding. If your doctor thinks you have an ectopic pregnancy, he or she will decide on the best treatment based on your medical condition and your future plans for pregnancy.

If your doctor suspects that you have an ectopic pregnancy that has ruptured, it is an emergency. You will need to have surgery right away.

All contraceptive methods reduce your risk of ectopic pregnancy. Those methods that stop ovulation (birth control pills, injections, vaginal ring, skin patch) reduce the risk the most.

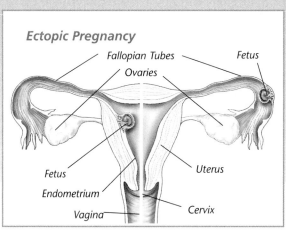

Ectopic Pregnancy

Fallopian Tubes

Ovaries

Fetus

Fetus

Endometrium

Uterus

Cervix

Vagina

A normal pregnancy (left) occurs in the uterus. An ectopic pregnancy (right) may occur in the fallopian tube.

Some women should not use birth control pills, including women who smoke and are older than 35 years of age. Women who have or whose family has certain health problems also should not use birth control pills (see box).

Although this rarely happens, the pill can cause severe illness in some women. The most serious problem is ***cardiovascular disease,*** such as blood clots in the legs or lungs, heart attack, or ***stroke.*** The risk is highest for women who smoke and are older than 35 years. They should not take the pill. When pill use is stopped, the risk is no longer increased.

Other rare problems may occur. They include:

- High blood pressure
- Gallbladder disease (in women already at risk for it)
- Liver ***tumors***

Most side effects are minor. But if you develop any of the symptoms listed in the box, see your doctor.

If You Miss a Pill

You may forget to take a pill once in a while. If you forget to take one pill, take it as soon as you remember.

Take the next pill at the normal time. It is okay if you have to take two pills on the same day. It is normal to feel a bit queasy if you do this.

If you forget to take two or more pills, use a backup method of birth control. Call your doctor or nurse and ask what you should do.

If you miss some pills, you may have some spotting or light bleeding even if you make up the missed pills. These side effects are not harmful.

If you have a 28-day pill pack and forget to take one of the last 7 "reminder" pills (pills without hormones), do not worry. Throw away the reminder pills you missed. Keep taking one pill a day until the pack is empty. You should start your new pack of pills on the same day of the week that you started your first pack.

Some women are afraid to take the pill because they have a family history of breast cancer. Most experts agree that women who have no other risk factors do not have an increased risk of getting breast cancer. These women can take the pill.

If your periods were not regular before you went on the pill, they may no longer be regular once you stop taking it. If you were able to get pregnant before you went on the pill, you should be able to when you stop taking it. It may take longer, though. Most women can become pregnant within 2–3 months after they stop the pill.

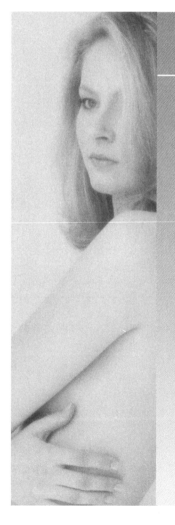

You Should Not Use Birth Control Pills If You Have:

- A history of blood clots in *veins* deep inside the legs

- A history of stroke or other disease of the blood vessels

- Active liver disease

- Unexplained bleeding from the vagina

- Breast cancer, past or present

- Lupus

- Uncontrolled high blood pressure

- Liver growths or cancer

- Heart disease

- *Diabetes* with eye or kidney problems

- Known *hypertriglyceridemia*

- *Jaundice* related to use of birth control pills

- Cancer of the endometrium or other known or suspected estrogen-dependent growths

- Known or suspected pregnancy

Warning Signs

If you are using birth control pills, visit your doctor if you have any of the following "ACHES":

A Abdominal pain

C Chest pain, cough, or shortness of breath

H Headache, dizziness, weakness, or numbness

E Eye problems, blurred vision, or speech problems

S Severe leg pain (calf or thigh)

Progestin-Only Pills

Some women may want or need to take another type of birth control pill that contains only progestin. This pill does not contain estrogen. It is called the progestin-only pill, or the minipill. It is not as effective as pills that contain estrogen.

The progestin-only pill is a better choice for women who have certain health problems—such as blood clots—and cannot take pills with estrogen. This method also may be the best choice for women who have had side effects with the birth control pill or who are breastfeeding. Because the progestin-only pill contains no estrogen, it does not cut down on the milk supply.

How They Work

Progestin-only pills contain only a small dose of progestin—about 25–70% of the amount in the combination pill. Minipills prevent ovulation in about half of a woman's menstrual cycles. They also change cervical mucus. The mucus thickens, making it hard for sperm to penetrate the cervix. Changes in the endometrium may play a role, too.

How to Use Them

The minipill comes in packs of 28 pills. All the pills in the pack contain hormones. It is important not to miss a pill. It is very important to take the progestin-only pill at the same time each day. It, therefore, may not be a good choice for people who have trouble staying on a schedule.

It is best to take the progestin-only pill early in the day. Taking it at bedtime could make it less effective. Cervical mucus protection is greatest between 4 and 20 hours after taking it.

You should use a backup method of contraception for 48 hours if vomiting occurs after taking a pill or if you are 3 or more hours late in taking a pill.

Health Benefits

Progestin-only pills do not offer the same benefits that pills with estrogen offer. But most people who choose the progestin-only pill do so because there are reasons they should not take estrogen. Progestin-only pills may offer some protection against:

- Cancer of the uterus and ovary
- Benign breast disease
- Pelvic infection

Side Effects and Risks

The progestin-only pill must be prescribed by a doctor. About 3–6 per 100 women will get pregnant while taking the progestin-only pill. The risk is increased in women who weigh more than 130 pounds. Women older than 40 years and women who are breastfeeding have lower failure rates because they are less fertile.

Possible side effects include:

- More bleeding or spotting days than with birth control pills that contain estrogen
- Prolonged or irregular bleeding
- Missed periods
- Headache
- Tender breasts

- Nausea
- Dizziness
- Acne
- Unwanted hair growth
- Weight gain
- Anxiety
- Depression

The progestin-only pill is not a good choice for some women (see box). Compared with pills that contain estrogen, the progestin-only pill increases the risk of:

- Ectopic pregnancy
- Ovarian cysts
- Vaginal bleeding

Progestin-Only Pills May Not Be a Good Choice If You:

- Know or suspect you are pregnant
- Know or suspect you have breast cancer
- Have undiagnosed vaginal bleeding
- Have trouble remembering to take birth control pills at the same time every day
- Have liver tumors
- Have acute liver disease
- Are taking certain medications
- Have active deep vein disorders

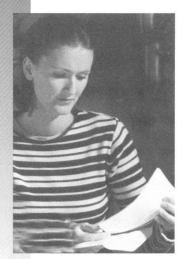

Emergency Contraception

Emergency contraception is a form of hormonal birth control that is used to prevent pregnancy after a woman has had sex without birth control or if a problem occurred with the method of birth control used (see box). It is a good option for women who have had unprotected sex and do not want to become pregnant.

The most commonly used method of emergency contraception is pills (also known as the "morning-after pill"). If there is some reason you should not take birth control pills, you may not be able to take emergency contraception. The IUD also can be used for emergency contraception (see box).

There are two types of emergency contraception pills. One type is combined birth control pills, which contain both estrogen and progestin. The other type contains only progestin and is safer for women who can't take estrogen. The progestin-only method may be more effective and is less likely to cause nausea.

Emergency contraception is a highly effective method of preventing pregnancy after unprotected sex. Pills must be started within 72 hours of having unprotected sex and will reduce

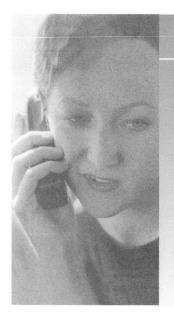

You May Need Emergency Contraception If:

- You didn't use any birth control.

- You had sex when you didn't plan to.

- A condom broke or slipped off.

- A diaphragm or cervical cap became dislodged.

- Birth control was not used correctly.

- You were forced to have sex.

There are many more reasons why someone has unprotected sex. No matter the reason, emergency contraception may be a good choice to keep from getting pregnant.

The Intrauterine Device for Emergency Contraception

The IUD can be a type of emergency contraception. The IUD must be inserted within 5–7 days of having unprotected sex. The presence of the IUD prevents the egg from being fertilized in the tubes or from attaching to the wall of the uterus.

A benefit of the IUD is that it can be left in for long-term use. The IUD may be a good choice if you cannot take birth control pills. The IUD is not a good choice for someone who needs protection from STDs.

the risk of pregnancy by at least 75%. The sooner emergency contraception is used, the more effective it is at preventing pregnancy. However, if you are already pregnant, emergency contraception will not work.

Doctor's offices, family planning clinics, and hospital emergency rooms may prescribe emergency contraception pills. If you have had unprotected sex, call your doctor's office right away. Be sure to tell them that you need treatment without delay. In some cases, your doctor can call in a prescription for you to your drugstore. You also can call the Emergency Contraception Hotline (888-NOT-2-LATE) to find a doctor who will provide you with a prescription.

Some doctors will give you an advance prescription for emergency contraception. This way, you will have it on hand if you need it. The sooner treatment begins, the more effective the method.

Widespread use of emergency contraception in the United States could prevent half of the 2.7 million unintended pregnancies and more than 800,000 abortions each year.

Emergency contraception should not be used instead of birth control on a routine basis. Regular use of a birth control method is more effective and has health benefits that emergency contraception does not have.

How It Works

The hormones in emergency contraception can prevent pregnancy in three basic ways, depending on where a woman is in her menstrual cycle, by:

1. Preventing ovulation

2. Keeping a fertilized egg from implanting and growing in the uterus

3. Blocking fertilization

This type of contraception only works within a short time after a woman has had unprotected sex. If emergency contraception is used later, it will not have any effect on the pregnancy or the health of the baby at birth.

How to Use It

Emergency contraception pills may be prescribed to you in one of three forms:

1. A specific dosage of regular birth control pills (either combination or progestin-only pills)

2. A prepared kit of four pills (contains estrogen and progestin) that may come with or without a pregnancy test

3. A package with two pills (contains progestin only)

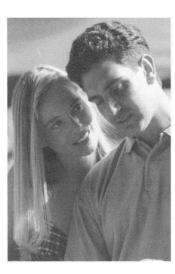

The kit with the pregnancy test and four pills also contains detailed instructions. You should read them first, then take the pregnancy test to confirm that you are not pregnant from a previous time you had sex.

If you take a pregnancy test and the result is positive, do not take the pills. Emergency contraception will not work if you are pregnant. Talk to your doctor. If the test results are negative, take the pills as directed to prevent pregnancy.

For the pills to work, timing is everything. The sooner you start taking them, the better. The pills are given in two doses. The first dose of pills must be taken by mouth within 72 hours of having unprotected sex. A second dose is taken 12 hours after the first dose. The number of pills in the dose depends on the brand of pill used.

After taking the pills, you may have some nausea and vomiting. The progestin-only pills cause less nausea and vomiting. The side effects will go away in a day or two. Your doctor may give you an antinausea medicine to take 1 hour before you take the pills. These medicines do not work as well if you take them after you feel nauseated.

If you vomit within 1 hour of taking either dose, let your doctor know right away. You may need to repeat that dose. If you vomit after 3 hours, you have absorbed enough of the dose and do not need to repeat the dose.

If you use emergency contraception pills within 72 hours of having unprotected sex, your chance of getting pregnant is greatly reduced. But there is still a chance that you could become pregnant. Using emergency contraception is not as effective as using birth control on a regular basis. Ask your doctor about a method of birth control that you can use regularly.

If you have sex after you use emergency contraception pills, you should use a backup method—such as a condom, spermicide, cervical cap, or diaphragm—until you have your period. If you were taking birth control pills before, you should keep taking the pills and use a backup method. If you have not had a period within 21 days of taking the pills, you should see your doctor for a pregnancy test.

Side Effects and Risks

Besides the typical side effects of nausea and vomiting, other side effects may include:

- Abdominal pain and cramps
- Tender breasts
- Headache
- Dizziness
- Fatigue

Any side effects will go away within a few days. Also, your next period may not be regular—it may be early or late, or light or heavy.

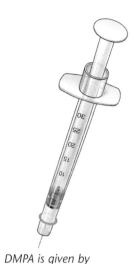

DMPA is given by injection.

Injections

One type of injection of hormonal birth control, called depot medroxyprogesterone acetate (DMPA), provides protection against pregnancy for 3 months. This means a woman needs only four injections each year. During the time that the injection is effective, she doesn't have to do anything else to prevent pregnancy. Another type of injection is given every month and contains estrogen as well as a progestin.

Injections may be good for people who find daily birth control methods inconvenient. Many women like the fact that this method doesn't need to be taken daily or put in place before having sex. It offers privacy to the user (there is no physical evidence of birth control).

DMPA injections also may be good for women who can't use combination birth control pills or IUDs. Injections can be used by women with seizure disorders. The level of hormones does not interfere with seizure medications, and the use of DMPA may reduce the frequency of seizures.

DMPA injections can be used when a woman is breastfeeding. They do not affect the quality of breast milk and may slightly increase the volume of milk. A woman can start DMPA injections after giving birth. Injections that contain estrogen should not be used by women who are breastfeeding.

When given correctly and on time, injections are very effective. However, if a woman becomes pregnant while using them, injections do not affect the pregnancy or the health of the baby. They do not protect against STDs. Use condoms for this protection.

How They Work

Injections are a type of hormonal birth control. They work in the same way as birth control pills because they:

- Suppress ovulation
- Increase mucus to keep sperm from entering the cervix
- Thin the uterine lining to prevent implantation

How to Use Them

A doctor or nurse must give the injection. It is usually given within the first 5 days of the menstrual cycle. This is to ensure that the woman is not already pregnant and to prevent ovulation during the first month of use. If the injection is given after that time, the woman should use a backup method for the next 7 days.

Side Effects and Risks

For every 1,000 women who use injections, only three will become pregnant during the first year. DMPA injections tend to cause irregular bleeding. During the first months of use, it is common to have irregular bleeding and spotting lasting 7 days or more. The frequency and duration of these episodes decrease with time. Eventually, a woman on DMPA may not have periods at all. About one half of women using injections for 1 year report no longer having periods; with further use, this occurs in three quarters of women. Women on the monthly injection containing estrogen have regular periods, as with combination birth control pills.

Injections may cause other side effects. These include:

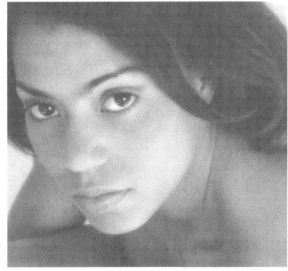

- Headaches
- Weight gain
- Worsening of depression
- Anxiety
- Acne
- *Hirsutism*
- Dizziness
- Decreased bone density
- Delay in return to fertility

On average, after a woman stops DMPA injections, fertility returns in 10 months. But for some, it may take much longer. If a woman knows she wants to become pregnant within the next couple of years, she should choose another form of birth control. The monthly injection allows rapid return of fertility, as with birth control pills. Some women should not receive hormonal injections (see box).

Health Benefits

There are many benefits of hormonal injections. They offer:

- Reduced risk of cancer of the uterus if used long term
- Possible protection against pelvic inflammatory disease
- Reduced pelvic pain caused by *endometriosis*
- The possibility of less painful periods
- Reduced incidence of ectopic pregnancy

Injections also may relieve certain symptoms of *perimenopause,* hot flushes, sickle cell disease, anemia, and seizure disorders.

DMPA Injections Are Not a Good Choice If You:

- Are pregnant
- Have unexplained vaginal bleeding
- Have breast cancer
- Have severe heart disease
- Have severe depression
- Have difficulty with injections

Vaginal Ring

The vaginal ring is a flexible plastic ring that is placed in the upper vagina. The ring releases both estrogen and progestin continuously to prevent pregnancy. The ring is worn for 21 days and removed for 7 days, and then a new ring is inserted. During the week it is out, a menstrual period occurs. A woman does not need to visit her doctor for insertion or removal of the ring, although it must be prescribed by a doctor.

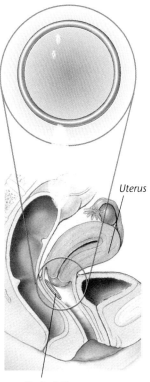

Uterus

Vaginal Ring

How It Works

The vaginal ring contains estrogen and a progestin. Just as with birth control pills, the vaginal ring increases the amount of these hormones in the body. These changes affect ovulation and other reproductive functions, such as thickness of cervical mucus and endometrium, and they make it hard for sperm to penetrate the cervix. Unlike the diaphragm or cervical cap, the ring does not cover the cervix. Pregnancy is prevented as long as the ring is in the vagina. When a woman begins using the vaginal ring, she should use a backup method of birth control, such as condoms or spermicide, for the first 7 days of use.

How to Use It

To insert the ring, squeeze the opposite sides of the ring together and push the folded ring into your vagina. This is all you need to do to place the ring in the correct position. Most women or their partners cannot feel the ring once it is in place. If you can feel the ring, it may not be placed back far enough in the vagina. Use your finger to push it back a bit further. You don't have to worry about the ring getting lost inside you because the cervix will block it from leaving your vagina.

After 3 weeks, remove the ring on the same day of the week and around the same time that it was inserted. To remove the ring, hold the rim and pull it out. Your period usually will start 2–3 days after the ring is removed. A new ring must be inserted 1 week after the last one was removed, even if your period has not stopped.

Although this rarely happens, the vaginal ring can slip out of the vagina if it has not been inserted correctly, while removing a tampon, or during a bowel movement. If the ring slips out, rinse it off and reinsert it as soon as possible.

You should be protected from pregnancy if the ring is out less than 3 hours. If it has been out for more than 3 hours, you may not be protected against pregnancy. In this case, you should use a backup method of birth control for 7 days.

If you lose the vaginal ring, insert a new one. Use the same schedule you would have used for the lost ring. If the vaginal ring slips out often, talk to your doctor. You may need to use a different method of birth control.

Health Benefits

In addition to preventing pregnancy, the vaginal ring may offer the same health benefits as combination birth control pills. The main difference is that you do not have to remember to take a pill every day, only to remove and replace the ring once a month.

Women who use the vaginal ring have a lower risk of cancer of the endometrium and ovary. The vaginal ring also reduces the risk of:

- Ovarian cysts
- Pelvic inflammatory disease
- Decrease in bone density
- Benign breast disease

The vaginal ring also helps relieve symptoms of polycystic ovary syndrome.

As with birth control pills, the vaginal ring can help keep your periods regular, lighter, and shorter. It also may help reduce menstrual cramps, and it lowers your risk of ectopic pregnancy.

Side Effects and Risks

The vaginal ring must be prescribed by a doctor. It is a very effective form of birth control. When it is used correctly, fewer than 2 in 100 women will become pregnant over 1 year.

Some women have side effects when using the vaginal ring. These may include:

- Headache

- Nausea

- Vaginal infections and irritation

- Vaginal discharge

- Breast tenderness

- Irregular vaginal bleeding

After a few months of use, many side effects go away.

Some women should not use the vaginal ring. This includes women who:

- Smoke and are older than 35 years

- Are pregnant

- Have certain health problems (see box)

You Should Not Use a Vaginal Ring If You Have:

- A history of blood clots in veins deep inside the legs, lungs, or eyes

- A history of heart attack or stroke

- Liver tumors or active liver disease

- Unexplained bleeding from the vagina

- Known or suspected pregnancy

- A history of heart attack, stroke, or other disease of the blood vessels

- Uncontrolled high blood pressure

- Diabetes with kidney, eye, or nerve problems

- History of, known, or suspected breast, endometrial, cervical, or uterine cancer

- Had jaundice related to birth control pills or during pregnancy

Skin Patch

The contraceptive skin patch is a small (1.75 square inches) adhesive patch that is worn on the skin to prevent pregnancy. The skin patch is a weekly method of hormonal birth control. Once a woman obtains a prescription for the patch, she does not need to visit her doctor to apply or remove it.

How It Works

The same hormones (estrogen and progestin) that are in birth control pills can be absorbed through the skin from a patch. With the patch, hormones are released constantly into the bloodstream through the skin. The patch prevents ovulation and changes the lining of the uterus. It also causes the cervical mucus to thicken, which makes it hard for the sperm to get through the cervix to the uterus.

How to Use It

A woman wears a patch for a week at a time for a total of 3 weeks in a row. During the fourth week, a patch is not worn and a menstrual period occurs. After week 4, a new patch is applied and the cycle is repeated, no matter when your period begins or ends. In this way, the patch works like the combination birth control pill. But instead of taking a pill every day, you put on a patch once a week. Although the patch is effective nearly right away, a backup method of birth control, such as a condom, should be used for the first week of your first cycle.

To use the patch, apply the sticky side of the patch to your skin. You may want to press on it for a few seconds to be sure that all of the edges are stuck firmly to your skin. Be sure to check the patch each day to make sure all the edges are still in place. To remove the patch, just gently peel it off your skin.

The patch can be worn on the buttocks, chest (excluding the breasts), upper back or arm, or abdomen. To ensure effectiveness, the patch should not be worn on other places on the

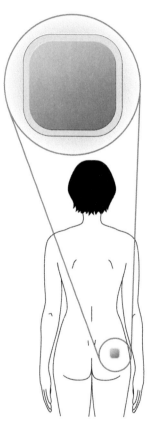

The skin patch can be worn on the buttocks (as shown), chest (excluding the breasts), upper back or arm, or abdomen.

body. Do not place the patch on skin where make-up, lotions, powders, or other skin products are applied. This can cause the patch to become loose and fall off. Do not apply the new patch to the same place on your skin each week. This may cause your skin to become red and irritated.

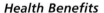

The patch is made to be worn for a week at a time. It should not come off during your regular activities, such as bathing, exercising, or even swimming.

If you forget to apply your patch, you should use a backup method of birth control for 7 days. Apply a new patch as soon as you remember.

If your patch seems loose or falls off and is off for less than 24 hours, try to reapply it or put on a new patch right away, and change the patch on the same day it was due to be changed. If your patch is off for more than 24 hours, apply a new patch right away and start a new 4-week cycle. You now have a new start day and a new day on which to change your patch.

Health Benefits

The contraceptive skin patch may offer many of the same health benefits as the vaginal ring and combination birth control pills. The patch can help keep your periods shorter, lighter, and more regular than typical periods. Women who use the skin patch have a lower risk of endometrial and ovarian cancer. The skin patch also reduces the risk of:

- Ovarian cysts
- Pelvic inflammatory disease
- Decrease in bone density
- Benign breast disease
- Polycystic ovary syndrome
- Ectopic pregnancy

Side Effects and Risks

The skin patch is a very effective method of birth control. When used correctly, fewer than 2 in 100 women will become pregnant over 1 year. Some women have side effects when using the skin patch. These may include:

- Skin irritation
- Breast tenderness
- Headache
- Nausea
- Menstrual cramps
- Abdominal pain

Some women should not use the skin patch. This includes women who:

- Smoke and are older than 35 years
- Are pregnant
- Weight more than 198 pounds
- Have certain health problems (see box)

You Should Not Use a Skin Patch If You Have:

- A history of blood clots in veins deep inside the legs, lungs, or eyes
- A history of heart attack or stroke
- Liver tumors
- Unexplained bleeding from the vagina
- A history of heart attack, stroke, or other disease of the blood vessels
- Uncontrolled high blood pressure
- Diabetes with kidney, eye, or nerve problems
- A history of, known, or suspected breast, endometrial, cervical, vaginal, or uterine cancer
- Had jaundice related to birth control pills or during pregnancy

Other Reversible Methods

In addition to barrier methods and hormonal methods, there are other forms of birth control a woman can choose. Some of these methods require a prescription from your doctor. Others do not require any devices or drugs. In choosing a method, think about what you feel most comfortable using. It's important to ask yourself what methods best fit you and your lifestyle. These methods do not protect against STDs. If you and your partner are not in a relationship with only each other, use a condom every time you have sex.

Intrauterine Device

The IUD is a small plastic device that is inserted and left inside the uterus to prevent pregnancy. Although there have been several types of IUDs, currently only two are available in the United States: the hormonal and the copper IUDs.

The IUD is a very popular method of birth control throughout the world. However, in the United States, fewer than 1% of women using birth control use an IUD. Many women are afraid to use an IUD because one type of IUD had problems and was withdrawn from the market in 1975. Today's IUDs are safer and more effective. The design has been changed, and doctors are careful about prescribing them to the right patients (see box). The IUD is more effective than most other forms of birth control.

The hormonal IUD must be replaced every 5 years. The copper IUD can remain in your body for as long as 10 years. As soon as the IUD is removed, there is no protection against pregnancy.

How It Works

Both types of IUDs are T-shaped, but they work in different ways. The hormonal IUD releases a small amount of progestin into the

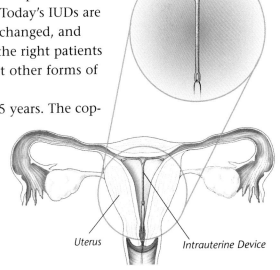

Uterus   Intrauterine Device

Do Not Use an Intrauterine Device If You:

- Are pregnant

- Have known or suspected pelvic cancer

- Have undiagnosed vaginal bleeding

- Have a known or suspected pelvic infection, including sexually transmitted diseases

- Have multiple sex partners

- Are at high risk for sexually transmitted diseases

- Certain liver disorders (copper IUD only)

uterus. This thickens the cervical mucus, which blocks the sperm from entering the cervix. It may make the sperm less mobile. It may make the sperm and the egg less likely to be able to live in the fallopian tube. It also thins the endometrium. This keeps a fertilized egg from attaching and makes menstrual periods lighter.

The copper IUD releases a small amount of copper into the uterus. A copper IUD does not affect ovulation or the menstrual cycle. It causes a reaction inside the uterus and fallopian tubes. This can prevent the egg from being fertilized or attaching to the wall of the uterus. The copper seems to work as a kind of spermicide. It prevents sperm from going through the uterus and into the tubes. It also reduces the sperm's ability to fertilize an egg.

How to Use It

A doctor or nurse must insert and remove the IUD. The IUD is easy to use. Once it is in place, you do not have to do anything else to prevent pregnancy. It does not interfere with sex, daily activities, or menstruation. You can use a tampon with it. Physical activity will not dislodge the IUD.

Your doctor will perform a routine exam to make sure you're able to use an IUD. It may include:

- Reviewing your medical history to determine any possible risks

- Performing a pregnancy test

- Taking a sample from your vagina and cervix to check for infection

You may not be able to use an IUD if you have:

- A uterine size or shape incompatible with the IUD

- A recent abnormal *Pap test* result

- Abnormal uterine bleeding

You may be asked to read and sign a consent form. Make sure you understand everything about the IUD to be inserted. If you have questions, ask your doctor.

The IUD is often inserted during or right after your menstrual period. The doctor puts the IUD in a long, slender plastic tube. He or she places it into the vagina and guides it through the cervix into the uterus. The IUD is then pushed out of the plastic tube into the uterus. The IUD springs open into place, and the tube is withdrawn.

Insertion of the IUD does not require *anesthesia*, although you may have some discomfort. Taking over-the-counter pain relief medication before the procedure may help. Sometimes a doctor will choose to use local anesthesia when inserting the IUD.

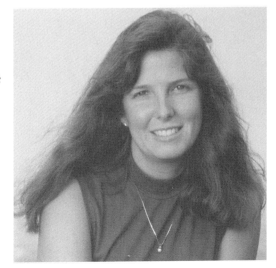

Once the IUD is inserted, the doctor or nurse will show you how to check that it is in place. Each IUD comes with a string or "tail" made of a thin plastic thread. After insertion, the tail is trimmed so that 1–2 inches hang out of the cervix inside your vagina. You will be able to tell the placement of the IUD by locating this string. The string will not bother you, but your partner may feel it with his penis. This should not interfere with his sexual feeling.

You may be asked to return for a checkup after your next period. You may also have a routine checkup about 3 months after insertion to check the placement of the IUD.

It is important to check the string regularly. To do this, you must insert a finger into your vagina and feel around for the string. You can do this at any time, but doing it right after your menstrual period is easy to remember. If you don't feel the string or if you feel the IUD, call your doctor. The IUD may have slipped out of place. Use another form of birth control until your IUD is checked.

A doctor must remove the IUD. Do not try to remove it yourself.

Side Effects and Risks

Fewer than 1 in 100 women who use the copper IUD will get pregnant in the first year of use. It becomes more effective with long-term use. The hormonal IUD is even more effective.

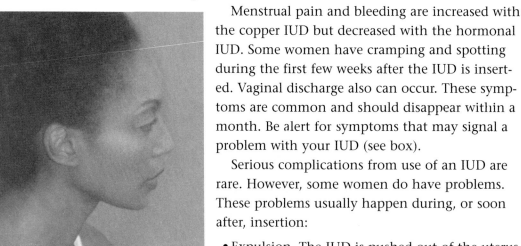

Menstrual pain and bleeding are increased with the copper IUD but decreased with the hormonal IUD. Some women have cramping and spotting during the first few weeks after the IUD is inserted. Vaginal discharge also can occur. These symptoms are common and should disappear within a month. Be alert for symptoms that may signal a problem with your IUD (see box).

Serious complications from use of an IUD are rare. However, some women do have problems. These problems usually happen during, or soon after, insertion:

• Expulsion. The IUD is pushed out of the uterus into the vagina. It happens within the first year of use in about 5% of users. This rate decreases

Warning Signs

These symptoms may signal there is a problem with your IUD:

- Severe abdominal pain

- Pain during sex

- A missed period or other signs of pregnancy

- Unusual vaginal discharge

- A change in length or position of the string

with length of use. It is more likely to occur in women who have not had children. If the IUD is expelled, it is no longer effective.

- Perforation. The IUD can perforate (or pierce) the wall of the uterus during insertion. This is very rare and occurs in only about 2 out of every 1,000 insertions.

- Infections. Infections in the uterus or fallopian tubes can occur after insertion. This may cause scarring in the reproductive organs, making it harder to become pregnant later.

- Pregnancy. Rarely, pregnancy may occur while a woman is using an IUD. If the string is visible, sometimes the IUD can be removed. If the IUD is removed soon after conception, the risks caused by having the IUD in place are decreased. If the IUD remains in place, there can be risks to the mother and fetus, including miscarriage, infection, or preterm birth. However, pregnancy may go to term with an IUD in place. If you are using an IUD and think you may be pregnant, talk to your doctor about your options and risks.

Natural Family Planning

Natural family planning is another name for the method of birth control that used to be called the rhythm method or "safe period." It also is called periodic **abstinence** or, more recently, fertility awareness. It isn't a single method but a variety of methods.

Natural family planning can be an effective way to prevent an unwanted pregnancy. In addition, knowing how to use these methods helps you understand more about your body's reproductive functions.

Whichever method you use, two things are essential:

1. Training by a medical professional or qualified counselor

2. Consistent use of the method

Natural family planning is very low cost and safe. It does not require drugs or devices. The success or failure of any of these methods will depend on your ability to recognize the signs of impending ovulation and to not have sex during the fertile period or to use another method, such as condoms, during that time.

You need to know your body well and you and your partner must be willing to follow the method. It can work only when you follow the method correctly at all times.

With natural family planning, the time during which sex is allowed is limited. Long periods of abstinence can be stressful for couples. Some couples may find it very hard to stick with this method.

Natural family planning is not as effective as most other methods of birth control. One in four women who use this method become pregnant. The method is not suited for some women (see box).

How It Works

Each method of natural family planning is designed to help a couple find out which days during the woman's menstrual cycle she is likely to be fertile or able to become pregnant. That way, the couple knows not to have sex during the fertile period

Natural Family Planning Is Not a Good Choice for:

- Women who should not get pregnant because of medical reasons

- Women with irregular periods who may not be able to reliably tell when they are fertile

- Women with persistent abnormal bleeding, vaginitis, or *cervicitis* (these make the cervical mucus method unreliable)

- Women who use certain medications (for instance, antibiotics, thyroid medications, and antihistamines) that may change the nature of vaginal secretions, making mucus signs impossible to read

- Women with certain problems unrelated to fertility (for instance, fever) that can cause changes in basal body temperature

to avoid a pregnancy. If pregnancy is desired, they will know the best days for conception.

Methods of natural family planning help the couple determine when ovulation is likely to occur. In most women, an egg is released almost 2 weeks before her next expected menstrual period. The egg remains able to be fertilized for about 24 hours after it is released. Sperm can live in a woman's body for 3 days or more. If the couple wishes to avoid a pregnancy, they avoid having sex during the fertile period, or the time around expected ovulation. The "safe period" includes those days in the menstrual cycle on which couples avoiding pregnancy can have sex.

Types

There are five methods of natural family planning:
1) basal body temperature method, 2) ovulation/cervical mucus method, 3) symptothermal method, 4) calendar method, and 5) lactational amenorrhea.

Basal Body Temperature Method. The temperature method of natural family planning is based on the fact that most women have a slight increase in their normal body temperature just *after* ovulation. Temperature readings also may be affected by fever, restless sleep, or varying work schedules.

A woman using this method takes her temperature every morning before getting out of bed. She then records it on a graph. In this way, she is able to detect the increase in body temperature that signals ovulation has occurred. For this method to work, a woman must take her temperature every day. A couple using this method does not have sex from the end of the menstrual period until 3 days after the increase in temperature.

Ovulation/Cervical Mucus Method. The ovulation method involves changes in how much mucus is produced by the cervix and how it feels. Women who use this method learn to recognize the changes that occur around the time of ovulation. To do this, a woman checks regularly for mucus at the opening of the vagina and assesses it for such changes.

For instance, for most women the vagina is dry for a time just after menstruation, then a sticky mucus appears. Just before ovulation, the mucus becomes wet and slippery. The last day of wetness, called the "peak" day, often occurs at the same time as ovulation. Just after the peak day, the mucus becomes thick again or may even go away, and the feeling of dryness comes back.

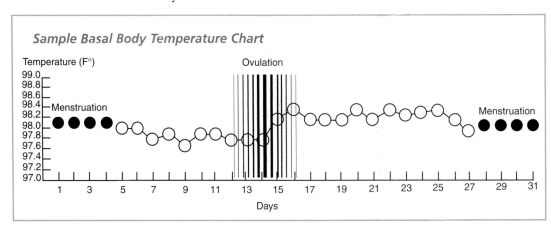

Sample Basal Body Temperature Chart

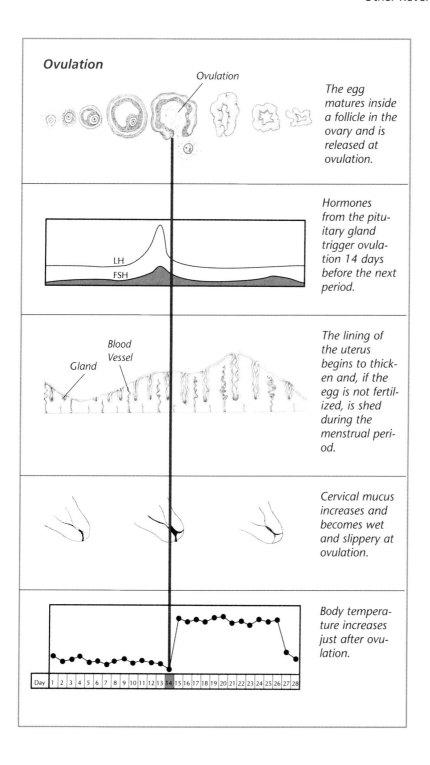

Ovulation

Ovulation

The egg matures inside a follicle in the ovary and is released at ovulation.

LH
FSH

Hormones from the pituitary gland trigger ovulation 14 days before the next period.

Gland
Blood Vessel

The lining of the uterus begins to thicken and, if the egg is not fertilized, is shed during the menstrual period.

Cervical mucus increases and becomes wet and slippery at ovulation.

Body temperature increases just after ovulation.

Day 1 2 3 4 5 6 7 8 9 10 11 12 13 14 15 16 17 18 19 20 21 22 23 24 25 26 27 28

The "safe" days (those days on which sex is allowed for couples avoiding pregnancy) are the 10 or 11 days at the end of the cycle and the dry days, if any, that occur just after menstruation. The fertile period (during which the couple should not have sex) starts with the development of the first signs of mucus and continues until 4 days after the peak day.

Although the days of bleeding are thought to be infertile, pregnancy can occur during menstruation. Mucus production may overlap the menstrual period. This overlap creates a place for sperm to live. An experienced user of the method is able to detect these changes.

The ovulation method has advantages over the temperature method in that it does not require the use of a thermometer and can be used by women whose menstrual cycles are slightly irregular. However, false readings may be produced by vaginal infection, sexual excitement, certain medications, and the use of lubricants for sex.

Symptothermal Method. The symptothermal method combines the temperature and ovulation methods. In addition to taking the temperature and checking for mucus changes every day, the woman checks for other signs of ovulation, such as:

- Abdominal pain or cramps
- Spotting
- Change in the position and firmness of the cervix

This method requires that you do not have sex from the day you first notice signs of fertility (mucus or wet feeling) until the third day after the increase in temperature or the fourth day after the peak day of mucus production.

The symptothermal method can be more effective than either of the other two natural family planning methods because it uses a mixture of signs. However, it has the same disadvantages as the other methods.

Calendar Method. The calendar method is also called the rhythm method. To use this method, a woman records every day of her menstrual cycle for 6 months. She then can calculate her fertile period by looking at the calendar (see box). Couples then avoid sex during the fertile phase. Because this method does

The Calendar Method

The first day of the fertile phase is found by subtracting 18 days from the length of the shortest cycle. To find the last day of the fertile phase, subtract 11 days from the longest cycle. In this sample, the shortest menstrual cycle in the past 6 months was 25 days. The longest menstrual cycle in the past 6 months was 35 days.

To calculate the fertile phase:
Subtract 18 from the shortest cycle (25 days) = 7
Subtract 11 from the longest cycle (35 days) = 24

This means the first day of the fertile phase is Day 7. The last day of the fertile phase is Day 24. If a couple is using this method to avoid pregnancy, they would not have sex during Day 7 through Day 24 of the woman's menstrual cycle.

not take daily physical changes into account, it is not as reliable as the others.

Lactational Amenorrhea. Lactational amenorrhea means a woman does not have her period because of a change in hormones caused by breastfeeding.

Lactational amenorrhea is a natural method of birth control. When a mother is breastfeeding without giving her baby any formula, lactational amenorrhea has a 2% pregnancy rate for the first 6 months postpartum.

This method loses effectiveness over time. A backup method may need to be used with it.

This method works better for older mothers than younger ones because older women are less fertile. Lactational amenorrhea does not protect against STDs.

How It Works

Ovulation and menstruation usually are postponed in breastfeeding women. These women have increased levels of a certain hormone, prolactin (which causes lactation). If a woman does not ovulate, she cannot become pregnant.

This method is most effective during the first 6 months of exclusive breastfeeding. Once vaginal bleeding occurs, the risk of pregnancy is greatly increased. Your doctor may ask you questions to determine your risk of pregnancy (see box).

Questions Your Doctor Will Ask Postpartum

- ❑ Have you had your period yet?
- ❑ Do you supplement feedings or allow more than 4 hours (during the day) or 6 hours (during the night) between feedings?
- ❑ Is your baby more than 6 months old?

If you answer "yes" to any of these questions, you have an increased risk of pregnancy.

How to Use It

For this method to work, a woman must be feeding her baby nothing but breast milk from her breast. The time between feedings should be no longer than 4 hours during the day or 6 hours at night. The baby should always be fed on demand. The more the baby feeds and the longer the suckling per feeding, the less likely it is that ovulation will return. Although feeding with formula on occasion may be fine, this may reduce the hormonal response in the mother and make ovulation more likely to return. A woman may begin ovulating before she has a period and will not know that she can become pregnant again.

Withdrawal

The withdrawal method prevents pregnancy by not allowing sperm to be released in the woman's vagina. It requires the man to take his penis out of the woman before he ejaculates. For this method to work, he must withdraw every time the couple has sex. Drawbacks are that:

- Sperm can be present in the fluid produced by the penis before ejaculation.
- Some men fail to withdraw completely or in time.

About 1 in 5 women who use this method become pregnant.

Sterilization

Sterilization is a procedure to prevent a woman from getting pregnant or a man from fathering a child. It is a very effective way to prevent pregnancy. The sterilization procedure for women is called tubal sterilization. The procedure for men is called vasectomy.

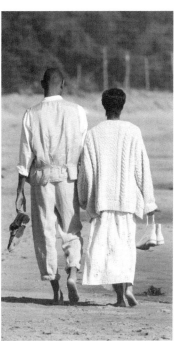

Nearly 1 of every 4 women in the United States relies on sterilization (of herself or her partner) for birth control. Sterilization is the most common form of birth control in the world. It is usually safe and free from problems. It is a permanent method of birth control.

Sterilization is an elective procedure. This means that it is your choice whether to have it done (see box). If you have doubts at any time—even after you've given consent—let your doctor know so that your doubts can be discussed. If you wish, the operation can be canceled.

Sterilization is an important decision. Although there is a slight chance that pregnancy can occur after the procedure, it should be thought of as permanent. You and your partner must be certain that you do not want any more children—now or in the future.

People may choose sterilization for a number of reasons:

- They may feel they cannot support any more children.

- They may not want to worry about birth control any longer.

- They may fear that a health problem could pose a danger to the mother's or baby's life.

When thinking about sterilization, remember that it is meant to be permanent. If there is any chance that you may want to have children in the future, think about other forms of birth control. You should also avoid making this choice during times of stress—such as during a divorce or after a miscarriage—and never under pressure from a partner or others.

Factors Affecting Choice of Method

The method of sterilization a man or a woman chooses will depend on physical factors, medical history, and personal choice. Sometimes previous surgery, obesity, or other conditions may affect which method can be used. The person should be fully aware of the risks, benefits, and other options before making a choice. You should also know the length of hospital stay (if any), cost, and time away from normal activities. Overall, vasectomy is easier and has less risk than female sterilization.

The decision should be carefully discussed with your partner. The final choice is yours, and the consent of others is not needed. The decision should be made with full knowledge of the procedure and the feelings of those close to you.

Sterilization can be done at any time. However, before the procedure you must comply with any legal requirements, including waiting periods. Discuss the rules and laws that apply in your case with your doctor.

You need to assume that sterilization will work and that it is not reversible. However, some people find that they regret their decision. If you are young when you make the decision to be sterilized, you are more likely to regret the decision. Others who have regrets may have made the decision when they were having marital problems or when they felt pressured by someone else to have the procedure. People often have a desire for sterilization reversal when they have a new partner.

If you change your mind after the operation, attempts to reverse the sterilization procedure may not work. The success of reversal depends on several factors, such as:

- The type of procedure

- How long it's been since the procedure

- Your age

- The length of the remaining fallopian tube

Reversing the procedure is expensive. It requires major surgery. Reversal procedures are rarely covered by insurance.

After tubal sterilization is reversed, rates of pregnancy vary widely. Also, the risk of problems, such as ectopic pregnancy, is increased. In men, the chances that a vasectomy can be successfully reversed also vary widely. To the couple, "success" usually is defined as having a child. But not everyone uses this definition when reporting success rates. Also, success rates never include people who were rejected for the operation.

Your doctor instead may suggest other options, such as *in vitro fertilization*. It is also expensive. An egg is removed from a woman's ovary, fertilized in a dish in a laboratory with the man's sperm, and then reintroduced into the woman's uterus to achieve a pregnancy.

After sterilization surgery, most women and men are able to return to their normal routine after a short period of rest. Side effects are minor and should go away in a few days.

The surgery does not affect either partner's ability to have or enjoy sex. It only prevents pregnancy. If a man and woman had a good relationship before the surgery, it should remain good. Many couples say that sex improves after sterilization because sex is more spontaneous without the need to use other forms of birth control.

Sterilization does not protect against STDs. Because they can no longer become pregnant, some women may become lax about protecting against STDs. Condoms should be used for this protection.

Female Sterilization

After sterilization, a woman no longer needs to use birth control or to be concerned about getting pregnant. It is effective right away. It does not affect a woman's sexual activity or menstrual cycle. If a woman used birth control pills before she had the surgery, though, it may take a while to return to her normal cycle. Although the cost for the procedure is higher than other methods, sterilization is cost-effective over the long term.

How It Works

Tubal sterilization works by surgically blocking or cutting the fallopian tubes. This prevents union of a sperm and egg.

How It Is Performed

Tubal sterilization can be done in different ways. If you are planning to be sterilized, you and your doctor will decide which method is best for you.

The two methods used most often are laparoscopy and minilaparotomy. Both methods have similar success rates and risks. Both can be done as outpatient procedures. This means you can go home the same day. Your doctor may have you stay in the hospital, though. Sometimes women have tubal sterilization right after the birth of a child. This is called postpartum sterilization and often is more convenient and faster than at other times.

If you have not been using a form of birth control, you may want to wait until during or just after your menstrual period to have this procedure. This timing will help avoid the chance that an already fertilized egg will reach the uterus after the operation.

On the day of your surgery, an intravenous line will be started. The intravenous line allows your body to receive fluids and medicines during the procedure.

You will be given pain relief (anesthesia). If a local or *regional anesthesia* is used, you may be given medication to help you relax before it is given. With epidural or spinal block anesthesia, an injection is given in the lower back, and the lower half of the body is numbed. You may be awake during the operation but will not feel any pain.

When *general anesthesia* is used, a tube may be placed down

New Option for Sterilization

Women who want a permanent method of birth control now have an option that doesn't involve surgery. With this method, a tiny springlike device is inserted through the vagina into each fallopian tube. This device causes scar tissue to build up in the tubes. This build-up blocks the fallopian tubes and prevents the sperm from reaching the egg. It takes 3 months for the scar tissue to grow, so women should use another method of birth control during this period. This device can be inserted in a doctor's office.

the throat to aid in breathing during the operation. If general anesthesia is used, you will not be awake during the operation. The type of anesthesia used depends on your medical history, choice, and the advice of your doctors.

Laparoscopy. First, anesthesia is given. The surgery then follows these steps:

1. A small incision (cut), about 1/2 inch long, is made in or near the navel.

2. A gas (in most cases carbon dioxide) may be passed into the abdomen to inflate it slightly. This moves the abdominal wall away from the organs next to it and allows the doctor to see the reproductive organs more easily.

3. The laparoscope is inserted into the abdomen. This device has a bright light and lens like a tiny telescope. This allows the doctor to see the pelvic organs. (Laparoscopy comes from the Greek words that mean "look into the abdomen.")

4. A device may be placed on the cervix to help move the uterus.

5. A smaller device is inserted to move and hold the tubes. The device may be inserted either through the laparoscope or through a second tiny incision made just above the pubic hairline.

6. The fallopian tubes are closed by tying, banding, clipping, or cutting them or by sealing them with electric current. The egg then cannot move down the tube, and the sperm cannot reach the egg.

7. The gas (if any was used) in the abdomen is withdrawn. The incisions are then closed, usually with one or two stitches, and covered with a small bandage.

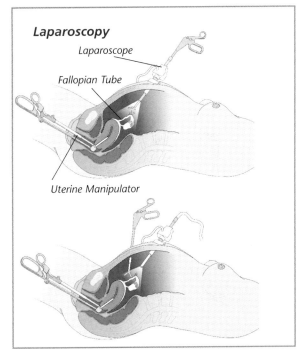

The laparoscope is placed through a small cut made below or inside the navel. A device (uterine manipulator) may be placed in the vagina to help move the uterus (top). *A second device may be inserted through another cut to move the organs into view* (bottom).

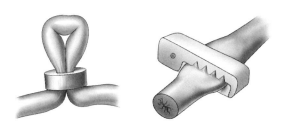

The fallopian tubes are grasped and sealed by using bands (left), clips (right), or electrocoagulation (not shown).

Minilaparotomy. A minilaparotomy is an incision made in the abdomen that may be only 1–2 inches long. Through this incision, the tubes are closed.

After anesthesia is given, a small incision is made in the abdomen just above the pubic hairline. The doctor may remove sections of the tubes and use surgical thread to tie the new openings shut, or the tubes may be closed with electric current, bands, or clips. A few stitches are used to close the incision, which is then covered by a small bandage.

Postpartum Sterilization. Almost half of the women who choose sterilization have it performed postpartum—while still in the hospital after the birth of their baby. Because the woman is already in the hospital and the new baby can be cared for in the nursery, this is a convenient time to have the procedure done. The surgery is easier to perform at this time, and it usually does not prolong the hospital stay.

In general, postpartum sterilization is done within 1–2 days after the birth of a woman's last baby. Many factors affect the exact time to perform it:

- Health of the mother just after the birth

- Health of the baby

- Time and personnel available for the procedure

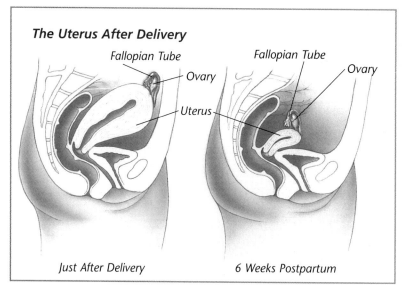

The Uterus After Delivery

Fallopian Tube
Ovary
Uterus

Fallopian Tube
Ovary

Just After Delivery   6 Weeks Postpartum

Just after delivery, the uterus is still enlarged, and the ovaries and fallopian tubes are pushed up just under the surface of the abdomen (left). At this time, the doctor has easier access to the tubes than at several weeks after delivery (right).

Talk to your doctor about it well ahead of time if you think you want to be sterilized after giving birth to your baby. It's a good idea to discuss it at your first prenatal visit.

In some cases, the procedure can be done a few minutes after the birth, with the same anesthesia used for delivery. If no anesthesia is used for the birth, the doctor will often wait a while before giving anesthesia and performing the operation.

After a woman gives birth, the still-enlarged uterus pushes the fallopian tubes up, just under the abdominal wall below the navel. In most cases, a small, 1/2- to 1-inch incision through the relaxed abdominal wall is all that is needed to bring the tubes into the doctor's view for the operation. There, the tubes can be grasped, then tied or cut. If you are having a cesarean birth, sterilization may be performed during the same operation soon after the baby is born.

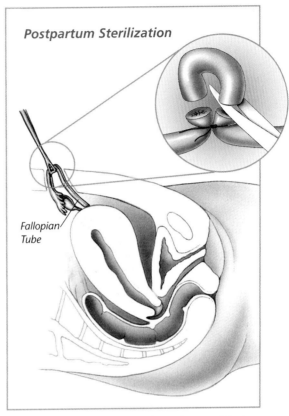

Postpartum Sterilization

Fallopian Tube

The fallopian tube is pulled through a small incision below the navel. A section of the tube is then closed off, and the section between the ties is removed.

After the Surgery

After surgery, you will be observed for a short time to be sure that everything is all right. Most women are ready to go home 2–4 hours after the procedure. You will need someone to go with you on the way home. You may feel some discomfort or have other symptoms that last a few days:

- Pain in the incision
- Shoulder pain
- Mild nausea from the medications or the procedure
- A scratchy throat (if a breathing tube was placed in your throat during general anesthesia)

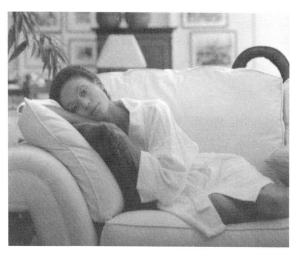

- Cramps
- Feeling tired or achy
- Swollen abdomen
- Gassy or bloated feeling
- Dizziness

Most symptoms usually go away within 1–3 days, and most women return to their usual routines a couple of days after surgery. After that time you may feel tired later in the day, have slight soreness over the incision, and have minor changes in bowel movements. Your discomfort often can be relieved with pain medication.

Contact your doctor right away if you have a fever or severe pain in the your abdomen. These could be signs of infection or other problems.

The incision should be kept dry for a few days to promote healing. A bruise around the incision, if present, will fade soon. If the incision appears red or swollen, your doctor should check to make sure there is no infection. After the incision has healed, a slight scar will remain. Keep in mind, you still need to see your doctor yearly for a routine exam.

Health Benefits

Sterilization offers a number of benefits. It does not affect a woman's menstrual cycle or sexual activity. However, women who used hormonal contraception will no longer have the benefit of shorter and lighter periods. Women who have been sterilized have a slightly lower risk of pelvic inflammatory disease and cancer of the ovary.

Side Effects and Risks

Sterilization is highly effective depending on the type of procedure. The risk of pregnancy with female sterilization is about 1 in 100 after 10 years.

Although the risk of failure is low, sometimes the sterilization does not work, and a woman can get pregnant. If you get pregnant after sterilization, it is more likely to be an ectopic pregnancy. See your doctor if you miss a menstrual period after the procedure and think you might be pregnant.

The surgery for sterilization is more invasive than other methods of birth control. All surgeries have some degree of risk, but serious problems are rare with sterilization. Each of the following problems occur in less than 1% (1 in 100) women who have this operation:

- Bleeding from the incisions made in the skin

- Bleeding inside the abdomen

- Infection

- Major side effects from the anesthesia

- Bowel or **bladder** injury

- Burn injuries to skin or bowel

Some women are at increased risk of problems with sterilization (see box).

Women at Increased Risk of Problems with Sterilization

You are at an increased risk of complications if you:

- Have diabetes

- Have a history of abdominal or pelvic surgery

- Have lung disease

- Have a history of pelvic inflammatory disease

- Are obese

Male Sterilization

A vasectomy should be considered permanent. This method can be used by men of any age. Overall, vasectomy is easier and less risky than most methods of female sterilization, and it costs less.

After a vasectomy, a man's sexual function does not change. He can still have an *erection* and ejaculate. Because sperm normally make up only 5% of semen, there will be little difference in the amount of fluid ejaculated. Sperm are still produced in the testes, but they are absorbed by the body.

For men who change their minds and want to father a child again, it may be possible to rejoin the tubes. This does not always work, however, especially if it has been several years since the operation.

Vasectomy does not protect against STDs. To protect against STDs, use a condom.

How It Works

Vasectomy involves cutting a man's vas deferens so that sperm cannot mix with semen. The tubes that carry sperm to the penis are clamped, cut, or sealed so that the ends do not join again.

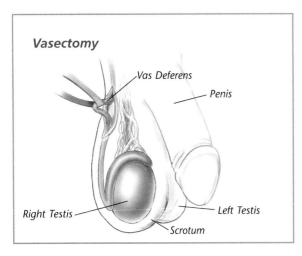

Vasectomy

Vas Deferens

Penis

Right Testis

Left Testis

Scrotum

In a vasectomy, the tubes leading from the testes to the urethra (the vas deferens) and tied, cut, and sealed to prevent the release of sperm.

How It Is Performed

Each side of the scrotum is cleaned with antiseptic and numbed with an injection of local anesthesia. One or two small openings are then made into the skin of the scrotum. Each vas is pulled through the opening until it forms a loop. A small section is cut out of the loop and removed. The two ends are tied and may be sealed with heat so that scar tissue will grow to block the tubes. Each vas is then placed back in the scrotum.

The procedure usually is performed under local anesthesia and takes no more than 30 minutes. It may be done in a doctor's office, clinic, or hospital.

Recently, some doctors have begun to use a "no-scalpel" technique for vasectomy. This procedure cuts the vas deferens the same way, but instead of making an incision, a special tool is used to puncture the scrotum in one place. No stitches are needed after the procedure. Patients have less pain afterward, and recovery time is shortened.

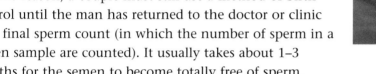

At least 1 day of rest usually is needed after the procedure. For 2–3 days after the operation, there may be some swelling and discomfort in the scrotum. If these symptoms last for more than a few days, or if there is a fever, severe pain, or other symptoms, the man should call the doctor.

A man can have sex again as soon as he feels comfortable. But unlike tubal sterilization in women, a vasectomy is not effective right away. Some sperm may still be in the tubes. For this reason, a couple must still use a method of birth control until the man has returned to the doctor or clinic for a final sperm count (in which the number of sperm in a semen sample are counted). It usually takes about 1–3 months for the semen to become totally free of sperm.

Side Effects and Risks

Vasectomy is simple and effective, and there are rarely any side effects. As with sterilization of women, though, vasectomy does not guarantee sterility. The failure rate is about 0.15%. It is more effective than female sterilization.

Some men may not be good candidates for vasectomy. These include men with certain **urologic** factors or increased risk of complications, such as:

- *Varicocele*
- *Hydrocele*
- *Inguinal hernia*
- Skins lesions on the scrotum or around the anus

Current research shows no increased risk of prostate cancer for men who have had a vasectomy.

Future Methods of Birth Control

Two methods of birth control are no longer available in the United States—the sponge and the contraceptive implant. Plans are underway to reintroduce modified versions of these products to the public in the future.

The sponge is a doughnut-shaped device. It is made of a soft foam that is coated with spermicide. It is pushed up in the vagina to cover the cervix. It acts as a physical and chemical barrier between the sperm and the cervix. Once the sponge is inserted, spermicide is released in small amounts for 24 hours. The sponge also absorbs semen before sperm enters the cervix.

Contraceptive implants are match-sized, soft plastic tubes that are placed just under the skin of a woman's upper arm. Implants release a low dose of hormones for up to 5 years. Insertion and removal of implants is done in the doctor's office using *local anesthesia*. A small cut is made in the upper arm and the tubes are inserted under the skin.

The Future of Birth Control

Birth control is a personal decision. There is not one method that will work for everyone. In the past 50 years, there have been many advances in the types of birth control available to women in the United States. There remains a need not only to improve existing forms of birth control, but also to develop new ones. New methods for women and men currently are being studied but have not yet been approved for use in the United States. Some of these methods are likely to become available in the future.

Special Needs

Every woman needs to consider her options carefully when choosing a method of birth control. But some women may need to think about additional factors in deciding what type of birth control is right for them. Teens and perimenopausal women, for instance, are at either end of the time in their lives when they have to think about birth control. Teens are just becoming fertile, and perimenopausal women are becoming less and less so. Unintended pregnancies happen most often in these two age groups, in part because some of these women don't think they can get pregnant.

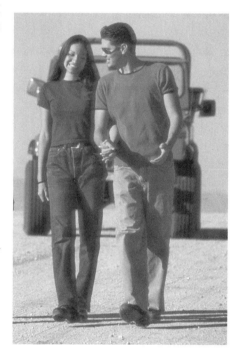

Breastfeeding women need to think about how a form of birth control might affect milk supply and the baby. Women with chronic health conditions may anticipate problems in pregnancy. They may wait to get pregnant until their health improves or they may need to avoid pregnancy altogether. This section considers some of these special needs and how they may be factors in choosing contraception.

Teens

In the United States, about one half of high-school women have had sex. Although teens in the United States are no more sexually active than teens from other countries, they are less likely to use effective birth control. Of teens who do use birth control, one third do not use it correctly.

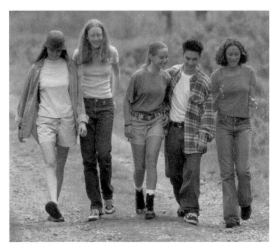

The pregnancy rates for teens, therefore, are higher in this country than in other industrialized nations. Each year, about 11% of women ages 15–19 years become pregnant. Of these pregnancies, 32% end in abortion, 14% in miscarriage, and 54% in live births.

The good news is that pregnancy rates among sexually active teens have decreased, and the use of birth control has increased. The percentage of women who use birth control the first time they have sex has increased as well.

There are many possible reasons why some teens do not use birth control. They may:

- Think they will not get pregnant
- Be afraid or embarrassed to go to a doctor or clinic
- Believe they must have a pelvic exam and are afraid of it
- Not believe they have access to birth control or know how to get it
- Worry about their parents finding out
- Be afraid that the doctor will share information with their parents
- Fear side effects of birth control
- Feel that birth control will make sex less spontaneous
- Think they cannot afford birth control
- Be afraid their partner will leave if they insist on using birth control
- Want to have a child

Most teens who are having sex do not want to have a baby. These teens should use effective birth control. They need to learn to use the method the right way and be sure to use it every time they have sex.

Seeing a Doctor

Many types of effective birth control require a prescription. This means that you have to see a doctor to get them. You may not need an exam at the first visit, though.

All sexually active women should have a well-woman exam once a year. This exam usually will include a:

- Pelvic exam

- Pap test

- Breast exam

- Physical exam (blood pressure, weight)

For the pelvic exam, you will be asked to lie on an examining table with your knees bent and spread, your legs raised, and your feet in stirrups. This position allows the doctor to check the outside of your abdomen with one hand and the inside of your vagina with the other.

The doctor inserts one or two fingers of one hand into the vagina and reaches up to the cervix. The uterus and ovaries can be moved from the inside with this hand while the other hand presses on the abdomen from the outside. In this way, the doctor can tell the size, position, and shape of these organs and may be able to detect tumors or cysts.

If a teen is very nervous about the pelvic exam, the doctor may put it off, even if she has chosen hormonal methods of birth control.

During the pelvic exam, your doctor may perform a Pap test. In this test, a few cells are taken from the cervix and vagina with a cotton swab or applicator. This is not painful. The sample will be examined in a lab for early signs of abnormal cells. Such abnormal cells could be precancerous or could signal cancer at an early stage. Sexually active

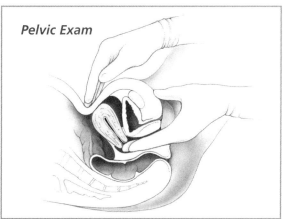

Pelvic Exam

For the pelvic exam, your doctor may check your abdomen, pelvis, and vagina.

women should have a Pap test once a year. Your doctor also will examine your breasts to check for cysts or lumps.

Many states give minors the right to make choices about birth control without their parents' consent. A teen should ask her doctor or nurse if the visit will be kept confidential. If a teen is using her parents' health insurance, she may not be able to hide the fact that she saw a doctor about something. If she talks about birth control with her primary care physician at the time of another visit, her parents may not find out. But if she tries to pay for birth control pills through insurance, her parents may find out. Often, the best way for a teen to maintain confidentiality and to afford birth control is to go to a publicly funded clinic. Some clinics may provide free birth control.

Some parents may be afraid that their daughter is at risk for pregnancy and may want her to use a long-term birth control method, such as injections. If the teen does not want to use birth control, she has the right to reject it.

Combination Birth Control Pills

Combination birth control pills are the most popular choice of birth control because they are so effective at preventing pregnancy and they have so many health benefits that appeal to teens, including:

- Regular periods
- Lighter menstrual flow
- Decreased incidence of menstrual pain
- Effective treatment for acne

Long-term use of this method provides other health benefits (see "Combination Pills," under "Methods of Birth Control").

Some teens are afraid to take the pill because they have heard stories about side effects or major risks. Teen fears related to the pill include:

- Weight gain
- Irregular bleeding
- No period

- Blood clots

- Cancer

- Stroke

- Problems with infertility

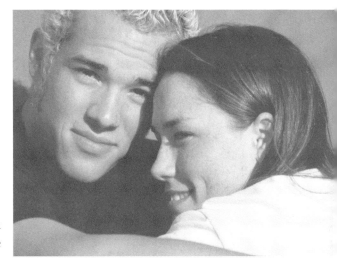

Most of these fears are unfounded, especially for teens. People believe many myths about the pill. Find out more about it before you rule it out (see "Combination Pills," under "Methods of Birth Control").

In order for the pill to be effective, you have to take it every day. You should take it at the same time every day. Tying the pill to a daily activity, like brushing your teeth, may help. If you miss pills and have sex, you could get pregnant.

The biggest problem with this method is taking the pill consistently. Teens miss doses more often than adults do. A teen may end a relationship and stop taking the pill. But if she starts another relationship, she is no longer protected from pregnancy. If you have been sexually active, you are likely to be so again. You should stay on the pill. Even if you do not have sex, you can benefit from regular menstrual cycles and other protective qualities. Do not stop taking the pill until you talk with your doctor.

You may have heard that you can't smoke and take the pill. If you smoke, you should try to quit. Smoking causes all sorts of health problems and complications. But if you smoke and are younger than 35 years, you can still take the pill. As a teen, your risk of cardiovascular disease is very low. A teen who smokes and is on the pill faces fewer risks than any woman carrying a pregnancy to term.

Besides combination pills, progestin-only pills are available. These pills are most often taken by breastfeeding women or women who can't take combination pills. They are rarely prescribed to teens, in part because the pills must be taken at the same time every day.

Other Methods

If you have trouble remembering to take the pill, you need to consider other choices of birth control. Methods like vaginal rings and injections do not require you to remember to do something every day. They may be a good choice for women who:

- Have had one or more pregnancies while using combination pills

- Have stopped using combination pills

- Are at high risk for forgetting to take their pills

- Do not want anyone to find out they are using birth control

These methods don't require you to do anything just before you have sex to prevent pregnancy. For more information, see "Injections," and "Vaginal Ring," under "Methods of Birth Control."

Injections of depot medroxyprogesterone acetate (DMPA) are linked with *bone loss* in teens. Injections provide a very private form of birth control, however. The vaginal ring also is a very private form of birth control, but a partner may feel it during sex.

Barrier methods—such as the diaphragm, cervical cap, or condom—can be very effective. But in order for them to work, the user must use the method correctly every time she has sex. Using condoms has the added advantage of protecting against sexually transmitted diseases (STDs). For more information, see "Barrier Methods," under "Methods of Birth Control."

In some cases, the intrauterine device (IUD) may be used by teens. If a woman has more than one partner, however, or if her partner has had sex with anyone else, she should not use an IUD unless she also uses a condom because the IUD does not protect against STDs.

Natural family planning is not a good choice for teens. It requires a lot of involvement from both partners and sometimes extended periods without sex.

Emergency Contraception

Emergency contraception is a form of hormonal birth control that is used to prevent pregnancy after a woman has had sex without birth control or after the method used has failed. Teens should be aware of emergency contraception and seek it out if they need it.

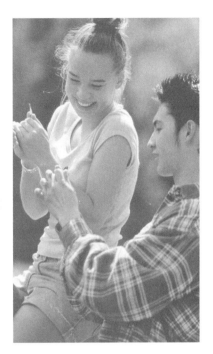

Emergency contraception should not be used instead of birth control on a routine basis. Regular use of a birth control method is more effective and has health benefits that emergency contraception does not have.

Some doctors will provide a prescription for emergency contraception before it is needed. This can be especially helpful with teens. For more information, see "Emergency Contraception," under "Methods of Birth Control."

Sexually Transmitted Diseases

Teens tend to underestimate their possible risk of infection with STDs. Every year, 4 million teens are infected with an STD.

Many teens practice serial monogamy. This means that when they are in a relationship, they have sex with only that person. After that relationship ends and they begin another relationship, they have sex with only that person. With every partner, they are exposed both to that person and to everyone else that person has had sex with in the past.

When a woman is using a hormonal method of birth control, she is less likely to use condoms, because she doesn't need them to prevent pregnancy. But hormonal methods do not protect against STDs. It is important for teens to use condoms every time they have sex (see box, "How to Use a Condom," under "Methods of Birth Control.").

Sometimes teens have oral or anal sex to avoid pregnancy. If you are having oral or anal sex, you need to use a condom to protect against STDs.

Breastfeeding Women

When you are breastfeeding, you are less likely to get pregnant. You may not ovulate or have your period for as long as you breastfeed (see "Lactational Amenorrhea," under "Methods of Birth Control"). To become pregnant, ovulation must occur.

It's best not to rely on breastfeeding as birth control, though. Because women's periods return at different times after delivery, it is hard to predict when you will begin to ovulate again. You could get pregnant before you even know you are fertile. If you are not ready for another baby right away, talk to your doctor about which method of birth control is good for you. What you were using before pregnancy might not be a good choice now.

Combination birth control pills contain the hormones estrogen and progestin. Estrogen can cut down on your milk supply. Women who want to continue nursing for as long as possible should not use contraceptives that contain estrogen. Progestin-only methods (such as the minipill or injections) or barrier methods (such as condoms) may be better choices for women who are breastfeeding (see box).

Birth Control for Breastfeeding Women

Hormonal Birth Control

- Progestin-only pills

- Injections

- Combination pills (may interfere with breastfeeding)

Nonhormonal Birth Control

- Lactational amenorrhea

- Additional protection:

  —Latex condoms (prelubricated)

  —Other barrier methods (diaphragm, cervical cap)

  —Copper IUD

  —Male or female sterilization, if permanent birth control is desired

Perimenopausal Women

Your body changes at midlife. Around your mid-40s, you enter a transition phase called perimenopause. It is a time of gradual change leading up to and following menopause. After menopause a woman no longer has periods and cannot get pregnant.

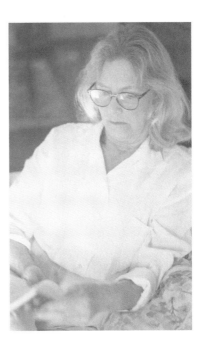

In general, perimenopause extends from age 45 to 55 years, although the timing varies among women. During this time, the ovaries produce less of the hormone estrogen. Other changes occur in your body as well. Because these changes happen slowly over time, you may not be aware of them.

Although your menstrual periods may become erratic as you get closer to menopause, pregnancy is still possible. Even having other signs of perimenopause, such as hot flushes, does not mean you can't get pregnant. About 75% of pregnancies in women older than 40 years are unplanned. You are not completely free of the risk of pregnancy until 1 year after your last period.

There are a number of factors to consider when choosing a birth control method at any age. Perimenopausal women should think about:

- Do I need to prevent pregnancy?
- Am I likely to develop health problems, such as brittle bones?
- Do I want to take preventive measures to maintain good health?
- Do I need to regulate my hormone level?

Combination birth control pills can be used by healthy, nonsmoking women up until menopause. They are a good birth control choice for perimenopausal women because they offer a number of health benefits:

- Control irregular bleeding
- Decrease bone loss

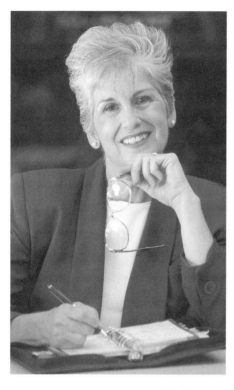

- Relieve hot flushes
- Decrease anemia
- Lower the risk of ovarian and endometrial cancer
- Lower the risk of ectopic pregnancy
- Decrease vaginal dryness

Some women may not be able to take combination pills, such as women who are older than 35 years and smoke or who have cardiovascular disease. Others may have trouble remembering to take a pill every day. But there are other birth control methods that are good for peri-menopausal women who are not at high risk for STDs, including the IUD, injections, and the vaginal ring. Barrier methods also should be considered. They are more reliable in older women because these women are less fertile.

Some birth control methods may not be as good a choice. Injections can affect menstruation. The long-term use of DMPA injections may lead to a decrease in bone mass, which may not be recovered before menopause.

The potential for an unintended pregnancy is high in this age group. No matter what you choose as your method of birth control, you may wish to talk with your doctor about emergency contraception (see "Emergency Contraception," under "Methods of Birth Control").

Women with Health Concerns

When a woman has a chronic medical condition, she has a lot more to think about when making decisions about birth control. Some conditions mean that a pregnancy at any time is dangerous. Other conditions may require medication that makes some forms of birth control less effective—or the birth control method may make the medication less effective.

If you have certain health conditions, you will need to ask yourself these questions:

- What is my risk if I become pregnant?

- If I am planning a pregnancy, what should I do to prepare for it? (For instance, should I change medication while trying to become pregnant?)

- What are the risks of taking my medication during pregnancy? What are the risks of *not* taking my medication during pregnancy?

- What is my risk if my pregnancy is unplanned or poorly timed?

- What are the possible bad reactions between my medication and birth control choice? Will the medication make the birth control not work? Will the birth control method make the medication not work?

- What role do things like level of exercise, diet, drug and alcohol use, and history of STDs play in my birth control choice?

Some methods may be safer and more effective than others. Also, some methods may offer health benefits. Barrier methods, such as condoms and a diaphragm, can be a good choice because these methods don't interact with medications. But in many women, the risk of pregnancy is of greater concern than the risks linked with more effective birth control. Therefore, when possible, your doctor is likely to recommend a more effective method.

Today's birth control pills have such low levels of hormones that most women can take them safely. Sometimes birth control pills even can help with some symptoms of a condition. But, there are women who would do better with nonestrogen methods, such as certain types of injections or an IUD. Most of these women have a condition that affects the cardiovascular system. Such a condition makes it dangerous for them to take estrogen. Because each woman's situation is different, you need to work closely with your doctor to figure out what method is possible for you (see boxes).

Women with certain medical conditions may be at an increased risk for complication during pregnancy. This may make choosing an effective method of birth control vital. Talk to your doctor about the best options for you if you have any of the following conditions.

High Blood Pressure

If a woman has chronic high blood pressure, she should try to control it through diet, exercise, and medication before becoming pregnant. High blood pressure can keep a fetus from receiving enough oxygen and nutrients to grow. Organs in the mother's body also may receive less blood than normal.

Birth Control Pills and Medical Conditions

Many women with chronic medical conditions are still able to take birth control pills. For some conditions, taking the pill poses no problems. For others, your doctor may prescribe the pill, but you may have to be watched carefully to make sure everything is going well. Sometimes certain formulations of the pill need to be used. If you have any of the following conditions, your doctor may consider prescribing the pill:

- Certain heart conditions
- Insulin-dependent diabetes
- Non–insulin-dependent diabetes
- History of *gestational diabetes*
- High blood pressure
- *Hyperlipidemia*
- Smoking (if younger than 35 years)
- Migraines (if not the classic type)

- Cancer (but not breast, endometrium)
- Human immunodeficiency virus (HIV)
- Immunosuppressive therapy
- Behavioral disorders
- Mental retardation
- Polycystic ovary syndrome
- *Prolactinoma*

Diabetes

If a woman has diabetes, she should have good control of the disease before she gets pregnant. She can do this through diet, exercise, checking glucose levels, and, if necessary, taking insulin or other drugs. At one time, the disease posed a major health threat to both mother and baby. Now it can be better controlled. Women who have chronic diabetes should get early care to help lower the following risks related to the disease:

- Miscarriage
- Birth defects (such as heart defects, kidney defects, and spinal problems)
- Pregnancy-induced hypertension (high blood pressure that appears in pregnancy)
- Hydramnios (too much amniotic fluid)
- Macrosomia (large baby)
- Stillbirth
- Respiratory distress syndrome (the baby's lungs don't fully develop)

Heart Disease

Heart disease affects about 1% of pregnant women. Half of all women with heart disease during pregnancy have congenital defects. The risk of problems during pregnancy depends on the type of defect and how severe it is. If a woman knows she has heart disease, she should talk to a doctor before trying to get pregnant. Both pregnancy and labor can be hard on the heart.

Lung Disorders

During pregnancy, the growing uterus alters the shape of the chest cavity. This, in turn, changes breathing patterns. One lung disorder—asthma—can deprive the mother and fetus of oxygen if it's not treated. Women with asthma should not stop taking their medication when they are pregnant and should be watched closely.

Birth Control and Medical Conditions

In women with the following conditions, use of progestin-only birth control pills or injections may be safer than combination pills. An IUD may also be a good choice for women with these conditions:

- Migraine headaches (not classic)
- Older than 35 years and smoke cigarettes
- History of thromboembolic disease
- *Coronary artery disease*
- Congestive heart failure
- Cerebrovascular disease
- Less than 2 weeks postpartum (except the IUD)
- High blood pressure
- Diabetes
- Lupus
- Hypertriglyceridemia

Kidney Disease

If the kidneys are scarred from a prior illness or don't function the way they should, it could affect pregnancy. The risks of kidney disease in pregnancy include miscarriage, high blood pressure, preterm birth, and stillbirth.

Lupus

Lupus is an autoimmune disorder. When a person has an autoimmune disorder, instead of protecting the body from disease, the immune system attacks the body's own tissues. As a result, organs can be damaged. Lupus can affect the whole body, including the skin, joints, kidneys, and nervous system. The disease tends to strike women during their childbearing years. During pregnancy, lupus increases the risk of miscarriage, preterm birth, and stillbirth. It can slow the fetal heart rate. In about one third of women, lupus gets worse during pregnancy.

Pregnancy Choices

No matter how in control of your fertility you try to be, sometimes things don't go as planned. You may stop using birth control in order to become pregnant and have trouble doing so. You may be using birth control and find that you have become pregnant when you don't want to be. Both of these situations can be very emotional and hard to handle. Pregnant women have to decide whether to carry a pregnancy to term or have an abortion. If they give birth, they have to decide whether to keep their baby or place it for adoption. Women who have trouble getting pregnant have to decide whether to pursue fertility treatments. They may also consider adoption—from the other side.

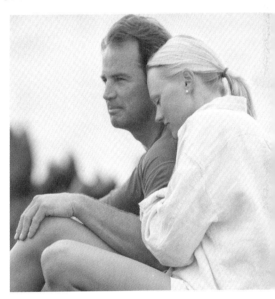

Infertility Treatment

About 15% of couples in the United States are infertile. Couples may be infertile if they have not been able to conceive after 12 months of having sex without the use of birth control. At this point, they may want to discuss it with a doctor. Many women take birth control for extended periods. When they stop taking it, they may have trouble getting pregnant because of age or for other reasons. Many of these women will be able to have children without medical help—it's just a matter of time. Women older than 35 years—whose natural fertility has begun to decline and whose reproductive time is more limited—may want to see a doctor after 6 months of trying.

A basic fertility workup can usually be finished within a few menstrual cycles. Find out what it will cost and what your insurance will cover. The workup will include:

- Physical exam

- Medical history

- Semen analysis

- Check for ovulation

- Tests to check the uterus and fallopian tubes

- Discussion of how often and when in your menstrual cycle you have sex

Basic Workup for the Man

A semen analysis is a key part of the basic workup. It may need to be done more than once. The sample is obtained by ***masturbation***. Sometimes it can be obtained at home. Sometimes it is obtained in a lab. Your doctor will give you specific instructions.

The semen sample is studied in the lab for:

- Number of sperm

- Shape of sperm

- Movement of sperm

- Signs of infection

Basic Workup for the Woman

The workup begins with a physical exam and health history. The health history will focus on key points:

- Menstrual function, such as irregular bleeding and pain

- Pregnancy history

- History of sexually transmitted diseases

- Birth control

Other tests, such as a Pap test and blood tests, may be done.

Some tests will be done to see if ovulation occurs. These include:

- Urine test (to measure luteinizing hormone, a hormone that causes ovulation)
- Basal body temperature (to detect a slight increase in temperature after ovulation)
- Blood test (to measure progesterone levels)
- Endometrial biopsy (to check for tissue response)
- Postcoital test (to examine the ability of sperm to enter and move into the cervical mucus just before the time of ovulation)

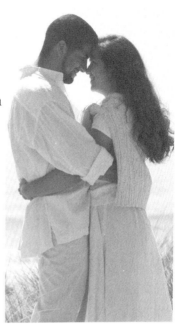

Some procedures may be done to look at a woman's reproductive organs:

- *Hysterosalpingography*
- *Transvaginal ultrasound*
- *Hysteroscopy*
- Laparoscopy

These tests check whether the uterus is normal and the fallopian tubes are open. The tests you have depend on your risk factors and symptoms.

Treatments

Medical treatment may be needed to help you become pregnant. If so, you should be aware of what is involved. Some treatments are expensive and require a great deal of effort from both partners.

If the cause of infertility is with one partner, then that partner can be treated. Medication may be given, surgery may be needed, or assisted reproductive technologies may be used. In some cases, treatments are combined to improve results. For instance, medication and insemination may be used at the same time.

Some of the treatments may include:

- Ovulation induction. The woman is given certain medications to cause ovulation to occur. She also can be given medication to increase the number of eggs released.

- Surgery. Surgery may be done to open tubes or repair other problems of the reproductive organs, such as growths or scarring.

- Assisted reproductive technologies. Some infertile couples require treatments that involve a lab using human eggs and sperm or embryos to help them conceive a child.

  —Insemination: Sperm is placed in a woman's vagina, cervix, or uterus by means other than sex. Sperm may come from her partner or a donor.

  —In vitro fertilization (IVF): Eggs from the woman and sperm from the man are fertilized outside the body in a lab. The fertilized egg then is placed in the woman's uterus to grow.

  —Gamete intrafallopian transfer (GIFT): A variation of IVF: a mix of eggs and sperm is injected into the fallopian tube during laparoscopy.

  —Intracytoplasmic sperm injection: One sperm is placed directly into an egg to fertilize it; fertilized eggs are placed in the woman's uterus to grow or frozen for later use.

  — Zygote intrafallopian transfer (ZIFT): A variation of IVF and GIFT; the egg is fertilized in a dish before placement in the fallopian tube.

Abortion

Abortion means ending the pregnancy by removing the developing embryo or fetus from a woman's uterus. Most abortions are done in the first 12 weeks of pregnancy. In some states, abortions may be done later in pregnancy, depending on the law.

The decision to have an abortion needs to be made as early as possible. The type of procedure used and some of the risks involved depend on how long you have been pregnant. The doctor can explain the stage of your pregnancy to help you decide. Your health also may play a role in your decision because some health conditions might pose a risk to a woman during pregnancy. You also may speak with a counselor. This is a good time to talk about your feelings and to ask any questions you may have (see the box).

Abortion is a personal decision. Because state laws about abortion can change, ask your doctor or counselor what the law is in your state. If you are a minor, state law may require that your parent(s) or guardian be notified or give consent or that you get permission from a court in order to have an abortion.

After the abortion you should be able to get counseling as well as recovery care. Your doctor may be able to refer you to a facility if he or she does not provide these services.

The Procedure

Induced abortion can be done in several ways. Some abortion procedures are done by surgery. Some are done with medication. The type of abortion you have depends on your choice, your health, and how long you have been pregnant. Care is provided for recovery and any problems that may occur. Most clinics also provide counseling.

Early surgical and medical abortions can be done safely in a doctor's office or clinic. Later abortions are performed in a hospital or clinic in most cases. The procedure for later abortions is more complex, takes longer, and carries more risk. It may depend on what facilities are available where you live. It also may depend on the state law.

Risks and Complications

Risks and complications of abortions relate to how long the woman has been pregnant. The earlier a woman has an abortion, the safer it is. Although an abortion is low risk, some abortions are a form of surgery. As with any surgery, problems, even death, may occur.

In most cases, having one abortion does not seem to affect later pregnancies. Little is known about the risk for women having more than one abortion.

Who Performs the Abortion?

Abortions are done by a doctor or other health professional who has been trained to do the procedure. Your own doctor may perform abortions. If not, he or she can refer you to someone who does. You also can find out about abortion services through your state's medical society, the local health department, or a family planning clinic.

The National Abortion Federation has a hot line that can provide information and guide you to providers in your area. The hot line number is (800) 772-9100.

Follow-up Care

You should have a follow-up visit after the abortion to make sure that you are healing as you should. You also should be counseled about birth control.

You may have feelings of guilt, regret, loss, or anger. You may feel relieved. All of these feelings are normal. This decision is easier for some women than others. A doctor's office or clinic can direct you to counseling to help you come to terms with this decision.

In most cases, after an abortion you can do any activities you feel up to doing. Ask the doctor who did the abortion if there is anything you shouldn't do.

Normal menstruation usually starts again from 4 to 6 weeks after an abortion. You can get pregnant soon after the abortion, so use birth control right away.

Adoption

If you cannot raise a child but do not want to have an abortion, adoption may be a good option. In an adoption, a child legally gets new parents. The baby will get a new birth certificate with the new parents' names on it.

If you choose adoption, prenatal care is as vital as if you were going to raise the child yourself. Be sure to start care early and see your doctor regularly.

You may have a mixture of feelings when the baby is adopted—anger, grief, a sense of loss, or relief. These feelings may last for a long time. They could return to you on the child's birthday, even years after the baby has been adopted.

Counseling can help you come to terms with this decision. The agency that provides the adoption service or a local family services agency may offer counseling.

The Process

Shortly after the baby is born, the birth mother (the woman who gives birth to the baby) signs papers that end her rights to the child and give her consent to the adoption. If the baby's father is known and he admits to being the father, he also signs consent forms. He may sign the papers before the baby is born.

After the adopting parents agree to accept the baby and have taken him or her home, they file legal papers asking to adopt the baby. A judge approves the adoption. After a waiting period (from 1 to 6 months, but sometimes longer), the adoption is final. Each state has its own laws about permission and consent and about the waiting period before the adoption is final.

Types of Adoption

There are two kinds of adoptions—open and closed. In open adoption, the birth mother and the adoptive parents know something about each other. They may meet and exchange names and addresses. The birth father also may be included. In a closed adoption, the birth mother and adoptive parents do not meet or know each others' names. Sometimes in a closed adoption, the files can be opened later. The laws in each state differ. Some protect the privacy of all involved more than others.

An adoption can be handled by an agency or, in some states, independently. Both agency and independent adoptions may handle open and closed adoptions. Check your state laws.

In agency adoptions, most agencies choose the adoptive parents after careful screening and study. Some agencies let birth mothers help choose. Babies may leave the hospital with the adopting parents or sometimes they may be placed in foster care.

In independent adoptions, babies are placed in the adoptive parents' home without an agency. Independent adoptions are legal in most states. They may be done through lawyers, doctors, counselors, or independent organizations. The birth mother may know who the new parents are. Before the adoption is final, the new parents and the home setting must be approved by the state agency that handles adoptions and by the court.

In an independent adoption, one lawyer can represent both the birth mother and the adopting parents. It is in the best interest of the birth mother, though, to hire her own lawyer. The adopting parents often are asked to pay for this. State bar associations can provide names of lawyers who handle adoptions.

One benefit of agency adoption is that the agency often provides counseling, support services, and follow-up after the adoption. There also may be fewer legal problems with agency adoptions. Agencies, however, may not allow adoption by single parents or parents over a certain age. Independent adoptions often have fewer rules and may have shorter waiting periods.

Financial Help

If you arrange an adoption through an agency, ask the agency what kind of financial help—both medical and legal—it offers. If you can't afford a private lawyer, you may be able to find legal aid. Legal aid often can be found at a university law school.

Most, if not all, states allow the adopting parents to pay the birth mother's legal and medical fees. Although these and other fees, such as counseling, often can be paid for the birth mother, it is not legal for anyone to make money from an adoption.

Resources

Finding quality information on birth control is the first step to making an informed decision. Your doctor should be your first source of information. He or she understands your needs and can help you decide the best method of birth control for you and your partner. Books, hot-lines, and health associations also can help you play an active role in preventing or planning a pregnancy.

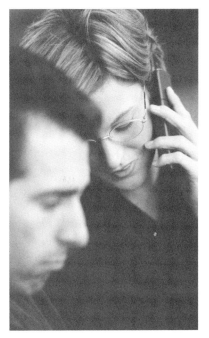

Books

Inclusion of a book in this list does not necessarily imply endorsement by the American College of Obstetricians and Gynecologists. This list is not meant to be comprehensive; the exclusion of a book does not reflect the quality of that book. The books listed below are usually available in public libraries or book-stores.

American College of Obstetricians and Gynecologists. Encyclopedia of women's health and wellness. Washington, DC: ACOG, 2000

Bell R. Changing bodies, changing lives: a book for teens on sex and relationships. New York: Times Books, 1998

Boston Women's Health Book Collective. Our bodies, ourselves for the new century: a book by and for women. New York: Simon & Schuster, 1998

Bullough VL. Contraception: a guide to birth control methods. Amherst, New York: Prometheus Books, 1997

Carlson KJ. The Harvard guide to women's health. Cambridge, Massachusetts: Harvard University Press, 1996

Epps RP. American Medical Women's Association. The women's complete healthbook. New York: Delacorte, 1995

Hatcher RA, Pluhar E, Zieman M, Nelson AL, Darney PD, Watt AP. A personal guide to managing contraception for women and men. Decatur, Georgia: Bridging the Gap Communications, Inc., 2000

Villarosa L. National Black Women's Health Project. Body & soul: the black women's guide to physical health and emotional well-being. New York: Harper Perennial, 1994

White EC. The black women's health book: speaking for ourselves. Seattle: Seal Press, 1994

Hotlines

Abortion Hotline
800-772-9100

AIDS Hotline (National)
800-342-AIDS (English)
800-344-SIDA (Spanish)
800-243-7889 (TTY)

Emergency Contraception Hotline
888-NOT-2-LATE

National Abortion Federation
800-772-9100

National Women's Health Information Center
800-994-WOMAN

Planned Parenthood
800-230-7526

Pregnancy Riskline
800-822-2229

Sexually Transmitted Diseases Hotlines
877-HPV-5868 (human papillomavirus)
(919) 361-8488 (herpes)
800-227-8922 (other sexually transmitted diseases)

Teen Helpline
800-637-0701

Health Associations

Alan Guttmacher Institute
1120 Connecticut Avenue, NW
Suite 460
Washington, DC 20036
Phone: (202) 296-4012
Fax: (202) 223-5756
Web Address: www.guttmacher.org

The American College of Obstetricians and Gynecologists
409 12th Street, SW
PO Box 96920
Washington, DC 20090-6920
Phone: (202) 638-5577
Fax: (202) 484-5107
Web Address: www.acog.org

American Medical Association
515 North State Street
Chicago, IL 60610
Phone: (312) 464-5000
Web Address: www.ama-assn.org

Association for Reproductive Health Professionals
2401 Pennsylvania Avenue, NW
Suite 350
Washington, DC 20037-1718
Fax: (202) 466-3826
Web Address: www.arhp.org

Centers for Disease Control and Prevention
1600 Clifton Road, NE
Atlanta, GA 30333
Phone: (800) 311-3435
Web Address: www.cdc.gov

Institute for Reproductive Health
Georgetown University Medical Center
3 PHC, Room 3004
3800 Reservoir Road, NW
Washington, DC 20007
Phone: (202) 687-1392
Fax: (202) 687-6846

National Women's Health Network
514 10th Street, NW
Suite 400
Washington, DC 20004
Phone: (202) 347-1140
Fax: (732) 249-4671
Web Address:
www. womenshealthnetwork.org

National Women's Health Resource Center
120 Albany Street, Suite 820
New Brunswick, NJ 08901
Phone: (732) 828-4503
Fax: (732) 249-4671
Web Address: www.healthywomen.org

North American Menopause Society
PO Box 94527
Cleveland, OH 44101-4527
Phone: (440) 442-7550
Fax: (440) 442-2660
Web Address: www.menopause.org

Planned Parenthood Federation of America
810 Seventh Avenue
New York, NY 10019
Phone: (800) 829-7732
Fax: (212) 245-1845
Web Address:
www.plannedparenthood.org

Appendix. Comparing Birth Control Methods

Method	How Used	How Obtained	Pregnancy Rates*
Spermicides	Applied each act	OTC	26%
Male condom	Applied each act	OTC	14%
Female condom	Applied each act	OTC	21%
Diaphragm	Applied each act; can be placed in advance	Prescription	20%
Cervical cap	Applied each act; can be placed in advance	Prescription	20% (40% for women who've had a baby)
Lea's shield	Applied each act; can be placed in advance	Prescription	15%
Combination pills	Must be taken every day	Prescription	3%
Progestin-only pills	Must be taken every day	Prescription	3–6%
Vaginal ring	Inserted monthly	Prescription	1–2%
Skin patch	Changed weekly	Prescription	1–2%
Injection (DMPA)	No action needed	Administered in doctor's office	0.3%
Injection (monthly)	No action needed	Administered in doctor's office	0.3%
IUD (copper)	No action needed	Surgical; placed in doctor's office	0.8%
IUD (hormonal)	No action needed	Surgical; placed in doctor's office	0.1%
Natural family planning	Couple diligence and training	—	25%
Female sterilization	No action needed	Surgical	0.5%
Male sterilization	No action needed	Surgical	0.15%

Abbreviations: DMPA, depot medroxyprogesterone acetate; IUD, intrauterine device; OTC, over-the-counter; STD, sexually transmitted disease; TSS, toxic shock syndrome; UTI, urinary tract infection.

*These rates are for typical use. This means that the method either was not always used correctly or not used with every act of intercourse, or was used correctly but failed anyway.

STD Protection	Side Effects/Risks	Reversible
Some	UTI, vaginitis, spermicide allergy	Yes
Yes	Latex allergy	Yes
Some	—	Yes
Some	Latex or spermicide allergy, UTI, TSS	Yes
Some (with spermicide use)	Latex or spermicide allergy, UTI, TSS	Yes
Some (with spermicide use	Abnormal bleeding or spotting, UTI, vaginitis	Yes
No	Headache, breast tenderness, nausea, irregular bleeding, missed periods, depression, cardiovascular problems	Yes
No	More bleeding or spotting days than with combination birth control pills, prolonged or irregular bleeding, missed periods, headache, breast tenderness, nausea, dizziness, acne, hirsutism, weight gain, anxiety, depression	Yes
No	Headache, nausea, vaginal discharge, infection, cardiovascular problems	Yes
No	Abdominal pain, allergic reaction on skin, breast tenderness, menstrual cramps, nausea, cardiovascular problems	Yes
No	Irregular periods, spotting, amenorrhea, headache, weight gain, worsening of depression, anxiety, acne, hirsutism, dizziness, slowing of bone growth, delay in return to fertility	Yes
No	Headache, weight gain, worsening of depression, anxiety, acne, hirsutism, dizziness	Yes
No	Heavy periods, irregular periods, painful periods, vaginal discharge	Yes
No	Irregular periods, vaginal discharge	Yes
No	—	Yes
No	Postsurgical complications	No
No	Postsurgical complications	No

Glossary

Abortion: The termination of a pregnancy before the embryo or fetus can survive outside the uterus.

Abstinence: Not engaging in sexual intercourse.

Acquired immunodeficiency syndrome (AIDS): A group of signs and symptoms, usually of severe infections, occurring in a person whose immune system has been damaged by infection with human immunodeficiency virus (HIV).

Amenorrhea: The absence of menstrual periods.

Anemia: Abnormally low levels of blood or red blood cells in the bloodstream. Most cases are caused by iron deficiency, or lack of iron.

Anesthesia: Relief of pain by loss of sensation.

Anovulation: Absence of ovulation.

Antibiotics: Drugs that treat infection.

Bladder: A muscular organ in which urine is stored.

Bone loss: The gradual loss of calcium and protein from bone, making it brittle and susceptible to fracture.

Breakthrough bleeding: Vaginal bleeding at a time other than the menstrual period; it sometimes occurs while taking birth control pills.

Cardiovascular disease: Disease of the heart and blood vessels.

Cervicitis: Inflammation of the cervix.

Cervix: The lower, narrow end of the uterus, which protrudes into the vagina.

Coronary artery disease: A disease in which the arteries that supply blood to the heart are narrowed by the buildup of cholesterol and other deposits in the walls of the arteries.

Cystitis: An infection of the bladder.

Diabetes: A condition in which the levels of sugar in the blood are too high.

Dysmenorrhea: Discomfort and pain during the menstrual period.

Ectopic pregnancy: A pregnancy in which the fertilized egg begins to grow in a place other than inside the uterus, usually in the fallopian tubes.

Endometriosis: A condition in which tissue similar to that normally lining the uterus is found outside of the uterus, usually on the ovaries, fallopian tubes, and other pelvic structures.

Erection: A lengthening and hardening of the penis.

Estrogen: A female hormone produced in the ovaries that stimulates the growth of the lining of the uterus.

Fetus: A baby growing in the woman's uterus.

General anesthesia: The use of drugs that produce a sleeplike state to prevent pain during surgery.

Gestational diabetes: Diabetes that arises during pregnancy; it results from the effects of hormones and usually subsides after delivery.

Hirsutism: Excessive hair on the face, abdomen, and chest caused by high levels of the male hormone androgen.

Hydrocele: A collection of fluid in part of the testicle.

Hyperlipidemia: High levels of any or all of the fats in the blood.

Hypertriglyceridemia: Too many triglycerides in the blood.

Hysterosalpingography: A special X-ray procedure in which a small amount of fluid is injected into the uterus and fallopian tubes to detect abnormal changes in their size and shape or to determine whether the tubes are blocked.

Hysteroscopy: A surgical procedure in which a slender, light-transmitting telescope, the hysteroscope, is used to view the inside of the uterus or perform surgery.

Immune system: The body's natural defense system against foreign substances and invading organisms, such as bacteria that cause disease.

In vitro fertilization: A procedure in which an egg is removed from a woman's ovary, fertilized in a dish in a laboratory with the man's sperm, and then reintroduced into the woman's uterus to achieve a pregnancy.

Infertility: A condition in which a couple has been unable to get pregnant after 12 months without the use of any birth control.

Inguinal hernia: A hernia—the protrusion of part of an organ or tissue through an abnormal opening—in the groin.

Jaundice: A buildup of bilirubin that causes a yellowish appearance.

Local anesthesia: The use of drugs that prevent pain in a part of the body.

Masturbation: Self-stimulation of the genitals, usually resulting in orgasm.

Menopause: The process in a woman's life when the ovaries stop functioning and menstruation stops.

Miscarriage: The spontaneous loss of a pregnancy before the fetus can survive outside the uterus.

Pap test: A test in which cells are taken from the cervix and vagina and examined under a microscope.

Pelvic inflammatory disease: An infection of the uterus, fallopian tubes, and nearby pelvic structures.

Penis: An external male sex organ that can become engorged with blood to increase its size, fullness, and stiffness.

Perimenopause: Around menopause; in the years leading up to menopause.

Perineal: In the area between the vagina and the anus.

Preterm birth: Born before 37 weeks of pregnancy.

Progesterone: A female hormone that is produced in the ovaries and makes the lining of the uterus grow. When the level of progesterone decreases, menstruation occurs.

Progestin: A synthetic form of progesterone that is similar to the hormone produced naturally by the body.

Prolactinoma: A growth in the pituitary gland that secretes excessive amounts of prolactin.

Prolapse: The falling or slipping down of an organ from its proper place.

Prostate gland: A male gland that produces most of the fluid for ejaculation.

Regional anesthesia: The use of drugs to block sensation in certain areas of the body.

Seminal vesicles: A pair of pouchlike glands on each side the of the male's bladder that secrete semen.

Sexually transmitted disease (STD): A disease that is spread by sexual contact, including chlamydial infection, gonorrhea, genital warts, herpes, syphilis, and infection with human immunodeficiency virus (HIV, the cause of acquired immunodeficiency syndrome [AIDS]).

Side effect: A usually unwanted consequence of a drug that happens in addition to its intended use.

Stroke: A sudden interruption of blood flow to all or part of the brain, caused by blockage or bursting of a blood vessel in the brain and often resulting in loss of consciousness and temporary or permanent paralysis.

Testes: Two male organs that produce the sperm and male sex hormone.

Transvaginal ultrasound: A type of ultrasound in which a transducer specially designed to be placed in the vagina is used.

Tumors: Growths or lumps made up of cells.

Urethra: A short, narrow tube that conveys urine from the bladder out of the body.

Urologic: Relating to the urinary tract.

Vagina: A passageway surrounded by muscles leading from the uterus to the outside of the body, also known as the birth canal.

Varicocele: Varicose veins in the scrotum.

Vas deferens: A small tube that carries sperm from a male testis to the prostate gland.

Veins: Blood vessels that carry blood from various parts of the body back to the heart.